Quality
Assurance
Handbook
for Veterinary
Laboratories

Quality
Assurance
Handbook
for Veterinary
Laboratories

James EC Bellamy & Dennis W Olexson

IOWA STATE UNIVERSITY PRESS / AMES

James EC Bellamy, DVM, PhD,
is professor of pathology,
Department of Pathology and Microbiology,
Atlantic Veterinary College,
University of Prince Edward Island,
Charlottetown, Canada.

Dennis W Olexson, BSc, ART,
is manager of diagnostic services,
Department of Pathology and Microbiology,
Atlantic Veterinary College,
University of Prince Edward Island,
Charlottetown, Canada.

Iowa State University Press
2121 South State Avenue, Ames, Iowa 50014

Orders: 1-800-862-6657
Office: 1-515-292-0140
Fax: 1-515-292-3348
Web site: www.isupress.edu

∞ Printed on acid-free paper.

First edition, 2000

Library of Congress Cataloging-in-Publication Data

Bellamy, James E. C.
    Quality assurance handbook for veterinary laboratories / James E.C. Bellamy and Dennis W. Olexson—1st ed.
        p.cm.
    ISBN 0-8138-0276-8
    Includes bibliographical references (p.).
    1. Veterinary laboratories—Quality control—Handbooks, manuals, etc. I. Olexson, Dennis. W. II. Title.

    SF756.3 .B46 2000
    636.089' 60756—dc21   00-022038

The last digit is the print number: 9 8 7 6 5 4 3 2 1

Contents

Preface   ix

1. Introduction   3

   Overview of a Laboratory Quality Assurance Program   4

   The Laboratory Quality Manual: A Framework for Quality

      Assurance   6

   Value of a Laboratory Quality Assurance Program   8

2. Quality Goals   11

   Analytic Error and Allowable Error   12

   Selecting Quality Goals   13

3. Mathematical Concepts for Quality Assurance   17

   Measures of Central Tendency   19

   Measures of Variation   19

   Data Distribution   20

   Confidence Intervals   20

   Accuracy, Precision, and Allowable Error   23

4. Monitoring for Quality   25

   Internal Monitoring—Quality Control   25

      Continuous (Interval or Ratio Scale) Measurements   25

         Selecting and Preparing Quality Control Materials   25

         Calculating Control Limits and Target Means   26

         Levey-Jennings Control Charts   26

         Which Control Rules and How Many Controls?   28

         Errors and Corrective Actions for Rejection Rules   30

         Calibrators, Controls, Reagents, and Instruments   31

         Definitive and Reference Methods and Reference Materials   31

      Categorical (Nominal Scale) Measurements   32

         Controls and Inspections   32

         Internal Audits for Quality Assessment   33

   External Monitoring—Proficiency Testing   33

5. Quality of Operations, Policies, and Resources 39

    Mandate, Services, Clients, Organizational Structure, and Budget 39

    Policies, Procedures, and Laboratory Management 40

    Laboratory and Equipment 42

    Financial Management 43

    Causes and Control of Preanalytic Variation 45

        Handling of Reagents and Supplies 45

        Handling of Specimens 46

            Random and Cyclic Biological Variations 46

            Diet-, Stress-, and Exercise-Induced Variation 46

            Variations from Technique of Specimen Collection 46

            Variations from Hemolysis and Intravenous Fluids 48

            Labeling Specimens 48

            Transportation, Centrifugation, and Storage 48

            Rejection of Specimens 49

            Records of Reagent and Specimen Handling 49

            Chain-of-Custody Considerations 49

    Laboratory Information Systems 50

        Main Features of the System 51

        Patient Identification 51

        Test Order Entry 52

        Specimen Identification and Tracking 52

        Interfaces with Analytic Instruments 53

        Entering Results into the System 53

        Reporting Results from the System 54

        Archives and Data Retention 54

        Quality Assurance and Management Aspects of the System 55

        Security of Laboratory Information 55

    Standard Analytic Procedures 55

    Standard Screening of Reports 56

    Interpretation of Laboratory Tests 56

6. Evaluating Laboratory Procedures 61

    Evaluating the Practicality and Potential Value 61

    Evaluating the Analytic Characteristics 62

        Within-Run Precision 63

        Reportable Range, Linearity, and Sensitivity 64

        Accuracy and Recovery 65

        Specificity and Interference 65

Run-to-Run Precision 66
Comparison-of-Methods Study 66
Correlation and Regression Statistics for Method Comparisons 67
Evaluating the Medical Characteristics 68
Medical Justification for a Test 68
Medical Characteristics of a Test 69
Reference Values 74
Documenting the Procedure and Informing Clients 77

7. Laboratory Choices and Point-of-Care Testing 79
Chemistry 79
Hematology 80
Coagulation 82
Cytopathology and Parasitology 82
Bacteriology, Histopathology, and Therapeutic Drug Analysis 83
Point-of-Care Testing 83

Appendix 1: Veterinary Quality Assurance Programs 85

Appendix 2: Conversion of Units 89

Glossary 91

References 95

Index 97

Preface

This book is intended as an introduction to the principles and procedures of quality assurance for veterinary laboratories. Laboratory test results are a significant component of the information used to make decisions in veterinary medicine. Errors in laboratory tests can lead to serious misjudgments in health management. Quality assurance procedures minimize errors and provide confidence in the validity of laboratory test results.

The book is a guide to, or outline of, the general components of quality assurance rather than a complete description of the various quality assurance methods that have been described for specific testing procedures. Veterinary laboratories vary considerably in the scope and types of tests they perform. Specific quality assurance procedures depend somewhat on the type of test being evaluated. Each laboratory or section can use applicable elements of generic quality assurance procedures, but often they must prepare and document formal programs that are tailored to their specific needs and activities. Many of the quality assurance procedures described in this guide may be in routine use in some veterinary laboratories; other laboratories may find helpful suggestions to improve the quality of their results. Although many of the quality assurance procedures described in the guide were developed for clinical chemistry, some of these are also applicable to testing in other disciplines.

This guide has been written both for practicing veterinarians and for professionals in larger commercial or institutional veterinary laboratories. Veterinarians who are doing laboratory testing in their practice require quality assurance procedures to have confidence in their test results. In addition, test results received from referral laboratories must be interpreted in light of other clinical information; quality assurance considerations are an essential part of valid test interpretations.

The guide begins with an introduction to the main components of a laboratory quality assurance program; a description of the laboratory quality manual, the main structure on which to build a good quality program; and a brief outline of the value of using quality assurance procedures. Other sections of the book discuss establishing quality goals; internal and external quality monitoring procedures; quality of operations, policies, and resources; evaluating new procedures; and quality considerations for point-of-care testing and office laboratories. Organizations offering veterinary quality assurance programs are listed in Appendix 1. Specific references are cited in the text and listed at the end of the book for supplemental reading. We would be pleased to receive critical comments or suggestions from readers for improving the guide for the future.

James Bellamy and Dennis Olexson
Atlantic Veterinary College
University of Prince Edward Island
-Charlottetown, PEI
Canada C1A 4P3

bellamy@upei.ca
olexson@upei.ca

Quality
Assurance
Handbook
for Veterinary
Laboratories

Chapter 1

Introduction

Every veterinary laboratory, whether it is a full-service commercial or institutional facility or a practitioner's office laboratory, can benefit from a quality assurance program. A laboratory quality assurance program has one overall objective: to provide confidence in the validity of the laboratory's test results and services. Veterinarians who receive timely laboratory results and are confident in their accuracy and reliability are more likely to make valid medical decisions regarding their patients. The public in turn will have increased satisfaction with the quality of veterinary health care.

The **quality** of all products and services is being increasingly emphasized by industry, governments, and the public. Concepts such as total quality management (TQM), continuous quality improvement (CQI), and the ISO 9000 standards are becoming commonplace in industry. In a similar way, attention to quality assurance is being focused on health-related diagnostic laboratories. The public expects the results from diagnostic laboratories to be accurate, reliable, and timely.

Human health laboratories for many years were each assumed to have policies and procedures in place to ensure the quality of their services and results. The quality of results from any particular laboratory depended mainly on the qualifications of their laboratory personnel, the internal quality control procedures that were used, and whether or not the laboratory participated in a voluntary external quality assurance program like that offered by the College of American Pathologists (CAP). Over the past two decades, the relatively narrow focus on the quality control of analytic procedures has expanded to a much broader look at quality assurance and quality management of all laboratory activities. In addition, countries have been developing regulations with systems of accreditation, certification, and inspection for human health laboratories to ensure the quality of their results. The Clinical Laboratory Improvement Amendments (CLIA) program in the United States is an example. If a human health laboratory does not sufficiently meet the CLIA standards, its activities can be curtailed or, in more serious cases, shut down.

For veterinary laboratories there are fewer regulatory controls. Laboratories that do studies on the properties and safety of chemicals in relation to human health or the environment (toxicity studies of new drugs or chemicals in animals, for example) often must abide by the principles of Good Laboratory Practice (GLP) formulated by the US Food and Drug Administration. In some countries, laboratories doing tests for the identification of certain infectious agents require certification by the appropriate government department for those specific test procedures (often in relation to export of animals or animal products). Otherwise, the scope of quality assurance procedures followed in veterinary laboratories doing routine diagnostic testing on animal specimens is controlled primarily by each laboratory.

With society's increasing demand for quality assurance of many services, veterinary laboratories have the opportunity to respond voluntarily and perhaps reduce the need for implementing as many regulatory and certification procedures as are required by human health laboratories. Voluntary quality assurance procedures developed specifically for the scope and types of testing done in each laboratory should be simpler to implement and more cost-effective than mandatory procedures. Several professional veterinary organizations have an interest in quality assurance of veterinary laboratories. For example, the American Association of Veterinary Laboratory Diagnosticians (AAVLD) offers a voluntary laboratory accreditation program for state, provincial, and university laboratories. This program encourages quality assurance in these laboratories, but the program is not open to commercial laboratories or to smaller laboratories in veterinary practices. Other veterinary organizations, such as the American Society of Veterinary Clinical Pathologists (ASVCP), are also concerned about quality assurance issues, but guidelines or recommendations for veterinary laboratories are not yet generally available.

Specific quality assurance programs available to veterinary laboratories are listed in Appendix 1.

Overview of a Laboratory Quality Assurance Program

The foundation of a laboratory quality assurance program is a desirable set of standards of quality—a set of **quality goals** for each laboratory test. These quality goals must be explicit and **measurable.** Quality assurance standards may arise from the laboratory itself, based on the expectations of its clients, from professional agencies, or from laws. Although there are few regulatory controls on quality assurance for veterinary diagnostic laboratories, quality results would be expected in any legal challenge related to decisions based on laboratory results.

Once the quality goals are defined, the quality assurance program works by repeatedly comparing the laboratory test results with the predetermined quality goals in order to identify and correct any deviations from the quality standard.

The components required to implement a veterinary laboratory quality assurance program effectively may vary somewhat depending on the activities of the laboratory, but in general they would consist of the following main items:

1. A laboratory quality manual to document laboratory quality.

2. Quality goals to provide direction to the quality assurance program.

3. Internal monitoring procedures to detect short-term changes in the quality of results.

4. External monitoring procedures to detect long-term changes in the quality of results.

5. Standard policies and laboratory procedures to meet the quality goals.

6. Research and development and test evaluation activities to assess the quality of new methods.

These general components of a quality assurance program will be similar for most types of veterinary laboratory, but the details of each of the above components would vary somewhat, depending primarily on the types of test procedures carried out. Each laboratory can develop a quality manual with a set of quality goals, can rigorously standardize its procedures, and can have problem-solving protocols and research and development activities to provide the solid base necessary for a quality assurance program. Most laboratories can avail themselves of an external quality assurance program to provide a periodic unbiased check on the accuracy of their procedures. Laboratories doing clinical chemistry, endocrinology, therapeutic drug monitoring, and aspects of hematology and serology, in which many of the analytic procedures are continuous-interval scale measurements, can use a range of quantitative methods for daily internal monitoring for errors. Laboratories that analyze mainly for discrete categorical results (e.g., cytopathology, histopathology, microbiology) can institute some internal control and auditing procedures to evaluate precision and accuracy but may depend more heavily on periodic external quality assurance programs to assess the accuracy of their procedures.

In addition to the six components outlined above, effective quality assurance systems depend on several common attitudes and ideas. First, the laboratory should be focused on the requirements of its users. Second, leadership in the laboratory should provide the vision for achieving quality, and the organizational structure of the laboratory should foster quality. Third, the laboratory should embrace problem-solving methods and be committed to continuous employee training and the involvement of all employees in planning.

To ensure not only that the laboratory quality goals are met over the short term but also that the quality assurance system improves in the long term, the components of a quality assurance program are implemented in sequence, as depicted in Figure 1.1. By implementing the elements of the program in this way, the quality goals, policies, and procedures are continuously evaluated and revised as necessary, resulting in continuous quality improvement.

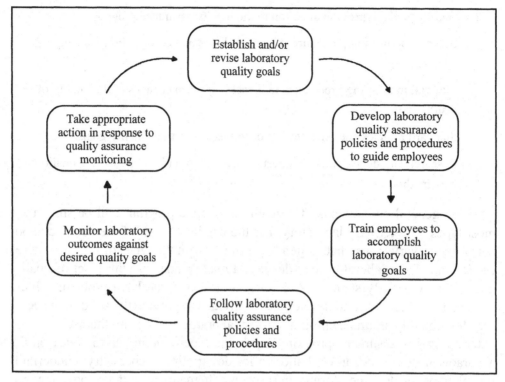

Figure 1.1. The cycle of activities for a laboratory quality assurance program to ensure continuous quality improvement.

The Laboratory Quality Manual:
A Framework for Quality Assurance

One general approach to the quality assurance of products and services developed by the International Organization for Standardization (ISO) is the ISO 9000 series of principles and elements of **quality management** that is now being used by many corporations. For applications specifically to services, the document ISO 9004 Part 2 contains information useful to veterinary laboratories interested in quality assurance.[2] The ISO 9004 document recommends a **quality manual** as an essential component of any quality assurance program.

We have adopted the view in this guide that the **laboratory quality manual** can serve as the framework and main instrument on which to build and maintain a good laboratory quality assurance program. The laboratory quality manual should describe the entire quality system of the laboratory. In addition to serving as a working guide to laboratory personnel for implementing and maintaining quality procedures, the manual can also continuously provide the documented evidence of quality for clients, accreditation agencies, or others. The contents of the manual would vary somewhat, depending on the scope of the laboratory, but a suggested table of contents for a laboratory quality manual is outlined in Table 1.1.

Table 1.1. Example table of contents for a laboratory quality manual

A. Quality goals
B. Internal quality control and audits
    1. Procedures
    2. Records
C. External quality assurance and proficiency testing
    1. Procedures
    2. Records
D. Quality of operations, policies, and resources
    1. Mandate, services, clients, organizational structure, and budget
    2. Policies, personnel, and laboratory management
        a. Hiring
        b. Orientation
        c. Training
        d. Continuing education
    3. Laboratory and equipment
        a. Description
        b. Records of maintenance, problems, solutions
    4. Financial management
    5. Information management
        a. Records
        b. Reporting
        c. Client communication
    6. Standards of handling and preanalytic sources of error
        a. Reagents and supplies
        b. Specimens
    7. Standard analytical procedures
    8. Standard screening of reports
    9. Standards for test interpretation
E. Evaluation of laboratory procedures
    1. Analytic evaluation of new laboratory tests
       Precision, range, linearity, sensitivity, accuracy, recovery, specificity, interference
    2. Medical evaluation of new laboratory tests
       Medical justification, medical characteristics, reference values
    3. Record of research and development activities

Developing a laboratory quality manual requires time and effort, but it will be useful in the laboratory as a central reference for all activities and will demonstrate the laboratory's commitment to quality assurance. Most laboratories will already have a standard procedures manual and records of internal and external quality assurance monitoring; if these items are integrated and the other sections listed in Table 1.1 added, then developing a laboratory quality manual should not be too difficult. Large laboratories doing a broad range of tests may find it convenient to subdivide a laboratory quality manual into several volumes separated either by discipline or activity, depending on the type of laboratory.

Value of a Laboratory Quality Assurance Program

Both the proprietors and the users of veterinary laboratories have a significant interest in the quality of laboratory results. Many decisions in veterinary medicine rely on the results of laboratory tests. Veterinarians who can be confident in the accuracy and reliability of results from a laboratory are more likely to make valid medical decisions for their patients; the clients of veterinarians in turn will have greater confidence in the quality of veterinary care. Laboratories that can assure users of the quality of their results are more likely to retain existing clients and gain new ones.

Although the scale and details of a quality assurance program may vary with the size and complexity of the laboratory operation, all veterinary laboratories can benefit. Large commercial and institutional laboratories may require a more detailed quality assurance program to avoid errors in a diverse range of analytic procedures. A more limited set of laboratory analyses done in a private veterinary practice would usually require a more modest quality program. The benefits of the quality assurance program are, however, similar in both settings.

Although a quality assurance program incurs an initial cost, this overhead is quickly offset by several cost- and reputation-saving benefits. Standard operating procedures often lead to more-efficient laboratory operations as personnel become familiar with the procedures. Standard protocols for error detection in a quality assurance program lead to earlier detection of analytic problems than do ad hoc trial-and-error approaches. The earlier error detection saves time and effort by the staff and maintains the laboratory's reputation. One or two serious laboratory errors can quickly sully the reputation of a laboratory, with potentially deleterious effects on its client base. Critical medical decisions rest on the results from laboratories that analyze animal specimens. Diagnostic, therapeutic, prognostic, and other important health management decisions may be based partly or entirely on laboratory results. A means to promote confidence in the validity of laboratory results is clearly advantageous. A good laboratory quality assurance program provides this assurance and thereby improves customer confidence and satisfaction.

In summary, a sound laboratory quality assurance program provides several important benefits to the laboratory and its clients:

- More efficient laboratory operations

- Earlier detection of analytic problems

- Increased confidence in the validity of laboratory results

- Improved interpretation of laboratory results

- Improved customer confidence and satisfaction

Chapter 2

Quality Goals

The **laboratory quality manual** should list a set of **measurable quality goals** for the laboratory. The general aim of a quality assurance program for a veterinary laboratory would be to provide valid and timely laboratory test results in support of effective medical decisions. Every laboratory would have a similar aim. But how can it be achieved, and how can its success be measured?

This general aim for quality can be more easily understood and achieved if it is expressed in more specific terms as a set of practical goals. To provide direction to a laboratory quality assurance program, each laboratory should develop a set of specific quality goals that the laboratory can pursue and measure to document its success at achieving quality. The particular quality goals selected by a laboratory will depend on the range and complexity of tests it performs, as well as on the history and current state of quality assurance in the laboratory. The quality goals should address accuracy, precision, timeliness, and any other factors that would improve quality.

Quality goals for accuracy and precision can be addressed in several ways, but each of them attempts to reduce analytic errors to the minimum required for the medical application of the test. The main sources of analytic error are **random error** (observed when one property of the same sample is repeatedly measured) and **systematic error** (the difference between the measured amount and the true amount). When combined, these sources of error determine the **total analytic error** of the method (Fig. 2.1).

In some instances the systematic error (bias) may be quite large, as in Figure 2.1A, and adds considerably to the total analytic error. In other instances the systematic error may be relatively small and unimportant relative to the size of the random error (Fig. 2.1B). In general, quality assurance programs are aimed at reducing the size of both systematic and random errors to that necessary for valid medical decisions. A change in size of analytic errors from those depicted in Figure 2.1A to those in Figure 2.1B would indicate improved accuracy with precision unchanged.

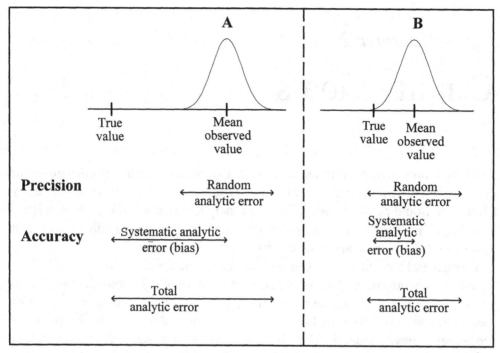

Figure 2.1. Types of analytic errors encountered in laboratory tests. (Adapted from Westgard et al.[3])

Analytic Error and Allowable Error

The goals for precision and accuracy should ideally be set in terms of the analytic error permitted to ensure a valid medical decision. For example, a medical decision level for hematocrit in dogs could be 0.36 L/L, such that a hematocrit of <0.36 L/L indicates a diagnosis of anemia. If clinicians at the same time generally believed that it is medically important that a true hematocrit value of less than 0.34 L/L should never be missed, then the precision and accuracy goals for hematocrit measurement must be such that a **reported value** of 0.36 has a **true value** somewhere in the range of 0.34 and 0.38. (See "Accuracy, Precision, and Allowable Error" in Chapter 3 for a more complete discussion of these concepts.)

To set these types of quality goals for precision and accuracy would require that the critical medical decision levels for each test be selected and the **allowable error** determined at each of the selected decision levels. In veterinary medicine this would be a difficult and time-consuming task. First, there are many animal species, and the medical decision levels for each test often differ not only among the various species but also often among the age, sex, and other subgroups of a species. Tests measured on continuous scales often have several decision points over the range of possible test results. In addition, medical decision levels for each test often vary with the use of the test (e.g., diagnosis, monitoring, prognosis). Another difficulty would be arriving at a consensus on critical medical decision levels for most tests; differences of opinion are common on these questions.

In the absence of agreed-upon medical decision levels, quality goals can be based on other criteria. One proposal suggests that the allowable error for a test should be the lesser of either 25% of the reference range or $\pm 10\%$ ($\pm 20\%$ for enzymes).[4,5] Another author suggests, based on human medical data, aiming for analytic precision levels that are 50% of the within-animal variation.[6]

Quality goals can also be set in terms of performance on an external quality assurance (proficiency testing) program. The goals can be described as limits to error in percentages, concentrations, or standard deviations. Reports from human medical laboratories indicate that the requirements for proficiency testing can usually be met if the internal laboratory precision is 25%–30% of allowable error limits for proficiency testing.[7,8] The assumption with these estimates is that the systematic error (bias) would be relatively low (as depicted in Fig. 2.1B). If the systematic error is high, then internal laboratory precision must be lower so that total analytic error is within the allowable error limits.

Selecting Quality Goals

With these latter considerations in mind, the sets of quality goals for our veterinary laboratory at Atlantic Veterinary College is described in Tables 2.1 and 2.2. These may serve as a guide for other laboratories. The goals for accuracy (the second column in the tables) follow closely those recommended in the Clinical Laboratory Improvement Amendments of 1988 (CLIA).[1]

The term "benchmark" in the second column of these tables can be defined as either the mean of all responses on a proficiency testing program or the mean of an acceptable reference method. The goals for internal laboratory precision (third column in the tables) are expressed as the expected coefficient of variation (CV) in a run-to-run precision study. This would be the same value as the **usual standard deviation** of a procedure expressed as a coefficient of variation. These precision goals are 25%–30% of the total allowable error goals in the second column of the tables. (The **within-run precision** generally would need to be approximately 50% of the **run-to-run precision** goals in order to meet the standards. See Chapter 6 for a more complete discussion of measuring within-run and run-to-run precision.) The last column of the tables indicates the turnaround time goals that our laboratory has to ensure that test results are provided in a timely manner. The accuracy goals are tested each time the laboratory uses an external quality assurance program (proficiency testing). The precision goals are tested regularly by internal quality control and/or internal auditing procedures to ensure that each precision goal is being met.

Table 2.1. Example set of quality goals for clinical chemistry and therapeutic drug monitoring in a veterinary laboratory

Variable	Accuracy Goals (Proficiency Testing)	Precision Goals (Analytical Precision)	Timeliness Goals (Turnaround Time)
Alanine aminotransferase	Benchmark ± <20%	± <5%	<1 hour
Albumin	Benchmark ± <10%	± <3%	<1 hour
Alkaline phosphatase	Benchmark ± <25%	± <6%	<1 hour
Amylase	Benchmark ± <30%	± <7%	<1 hour
Aspartate aminotransferase	Benchmark ± <20%	± <5%	<1 hour
Bilirubin	Benchmark ± <20%	± <5%	<1 hour
Calcium	Benchmark ± <10%	± <3%	<1 hour
Chloride	Benchmark ± <8%	± <2%	<1 hour
Cholesterol	Benchmark ± <10%	± <3%	<1 hour
Cortisol	Benchmark ± <25%	± <6%	<1 hour
Creatine phosphokinase	Benchmark ± <30%	± <7%	<1 hour
Creatinine	Benchmark ± <20%	± <5%	<1 hour
Gamma glutamic transaminase	Benchmark ± <25%	± <6%	<1 hour
Glucose	Benchmark ± <10%	± <3%	<1 hour
Iron	Benchmark ± <20%	± <5%	<1 hour
Lipase	Benchmark ± <30%	± <7%	<1 hour
Magnesium	Benchmark ± <20%	± <5%	<1 hour
pH	Benchmark ± <0.06 units	± <0.02 units	<1 hour
PCO_2	Benchmark ± <8%	± <2%	<1 hour
PO_2	Benchmark ± <10%	± <3%	<1 hour
Potassium	Benchmark ± <10%	± <3%	<1 hour
Protein	Benchmark ± <10%	± <3%	<1 hour
Sodium	Benchmark ± <6%	± <2%	<1 hour
Thyroid stimulating hormone	Benchmark ± <3 sd[a]	± <0.75[a]	<8 hours
Thyroxine	Benchmark ± <25%	± <6%	<4 hours
Urea	Benchmark ± <12%	± <4%	<1 hour
Digoxin	Benchmark ± <20%	± <5%	<1 hour
Dilantin	Benchmark ± <20%	± <5%	<1 hour
Phenobarbital	Benchmark ± <20%	± <5%	<1 hour

Note: The proficiency testing and analytical performance goals are those of the Diagnostic Services Unit, Atlantic Veterinary College, University of Prince Edward Island, Charlottetown, Canada. The criteria closely follow those recommended in the Clinical Laboratory Improvement Amendments of 1988 (CLIA).[1]

[a] sd represents standard deviation.

Table 2.2. Example set of quality goals for hematology, cytology, serology, histopathology, bacteriology, and parasitology in a veterinary laboratory

Variable	Accuracy Goals (Proficiency Testing)	Precision Goals (Analytical Precision)	Timeliness Goals (Turnaround Time)
Erythrocyte count	Benchmark ± <8%	± <2%	<1 hour
Hematocrit	Benchmark ± <8%	± <2%	<1 hour
Hemoglobin	Benchmark ± <8%	± <2%	<1 hour
Leukocyte count	Benchmark ± <15%	± <4%	<1 hour
Platelet count	Benchmark ± <25%	± <6%	<1 hour
Fibrinogen	Benchmark ± <20%	± <5%	<1 hour
Partial thromboplastin time	Benchmark ± <15%	± <4%	<1 hour
Prothrombin time	Benchmark ± <15%	± <4%	<1 hour
White cell differential	Benchmark ± <3 SD for each cell type	Within <3 SD for each cell type on internal audit	<1 hour
Cell identification	>90% agreement with benchmark	>90% agreement on internal audit	<1 hour
Cytologic diagnosis	>90% agreement with benchmark	>90% agreement on internal audit	<2 hours
Histopathologic diagnosis	>90% agreement with benchmark	>90% agreement on internal audit	<48 hours
Bacterial culture identification	>90% agreement with benchmark	>90% agreement on internal audit	<24/48 hours
Parasite identification	>90% agreement with benchmark	>90% agreement on internal audit	<1 hour
Serology (titers)	Benchmark ± 2 dilutions	± <7%	<6/24/48 hours
Serology (+ or −)	>90% agreement with benchmark	>90% agreement on internal audit	<6/24/48 hours

Note: The proficiency testing and analytical performance goals are those of the Diagnostic Services Unit, Atlantic Veterinary College, University of Prince Edward Island, Charlottetown, Canada. The criteria closely follow those recommended in the Clinical Laboratory Improvement Amendments of 1988 (CLIA).[1]

An example will help illustrate how the goals can be used to measure the quality of laboratory results. The accuracy goal, or total allowable error, for albumin (Table 2.1) is "benchmark $\pm$ <10%." If the peer group mean for albumin on our proficiency testing program was 19.6 g/L, we would want our result to be in the range of 19.6 $\pm$ <10%, that is, between 17.6 and 21.6 g/L. Our proficiency testing result for albumin was 18.4 g/L, which was ~6.2% from the group mean and therefore well within $\pm$ <10% of the benchmark. We could then feel confident that our albumin method and results were sufficiently accurate. Our internal precision goal for albumin is to have a usual CV of <3%. The goal is based on the estimate that it should be about 25%–30% of the accuracy goal. The quality control precision results on our albumin method indicate a target mean, plus or minus usual standard deviation, of 19.2 $\pm$ 0.54 g/L. This indicates a CV of 2.8%, which is within our 3% limit.

It is important to keep in mind that the quality goals are guidelines to be used in conjunction with an external quality assurance (proficiency testing) program. Goals based on specific medical decision levels, if available, may be preferable. The goals listed in Tables 2.1 and 2.2 are expressed as percentages, with the result that at higher concentrations of analyte a proportionally greater error will be acceptable. If it has been determined that, at a specific medical decision level, the allowable error for a valid medical decision is less than the stated percentage guideline, the existing quality goal may be replaced with the more rigorous one that is based on the medical decision level. However, if it has been determined that there is so much "normal" biological variation in the values of a variable that such a rigorous analytic precision goal has no value, the precision goal could be adjusted upward accordingly.

Quality goals for factors other than accuracy, precision, and timeliness may be necessary. A laboratory that has been using manual methods of recording and reporting information, for example, may have an additional quality goal of developing an electronic information management system to reduce both the number of transcription errors in laboratory reports and the time required for these activities. (Laboratory information management systems are discussed in Chapter 5.) The interpretation of test results is also important and can be evaluated by internal audits, external quality assurance programs, and client feedback questionnaires.

Chapter 3

Mathematical Concepts for Quality Assurance

Our understanding of health and disease in animals is in terms of the properties of animals and their environment. A **property** of an animal is any characteristic; blood type, body temperature, heart rate, number of fecal coliform bacilli, and serum glucose concentration are examples of properties. By measuring properties of animals and determining the relationships among those properties, we acquire the knowledge on which medical decisions are based. Diagnostic, prognostic, therapeutic, and health management decisions are all based on measured properties of animals.

To measure a property of an animal, the property must be applied to a **scale of measurement**. The scale of measurement must be considered when mathematical calculations for precision, accuracy, and test comparisons are used for quality assurance. There are four scales of measurement: nominal, ordinal, interval, and ratio (Table 3.1).

Nominal scale measurement involves assigning an object to a category according to whether or not it possesses a property. The categories are not continuous; they are distinct. Blood type, for example, could be measured as one of three distinct categories—type A, type B, or type O. **Ordinal scale** measurement involves assigning an object to a category according to the degree to which an object possesses a property. The categories are continuous; there is order to the categories. Scoring spherocytes on a blood smear on a four-point scale from 0 to +++ is an example of ordinal scale measurement. Although there is order in the categories of an ordinal scale, the intervals between each category are not necessarily the same size. In this example, the difference between 0 and + may be smaller or larger than the difference between ++ and +++. A continuous measurement scale with intervals of equal size is called an **interval scale**. In the Fahrenheit temperature scale, the interval between 10°F and 11°F is the same as that between 17°F and 18°F.

Table 3.1. Properties, scales of measurement, and statistics

Property	Units of Measurement	Scale of Measurement	Descriptive Statistics
Blood type	Type A, Type B, Type O	Nominal	Mode
Spherocytic red cells	0, +, ++, +++	Ordinal	Mode, median, percentiles
Body temperature	° Fahrenheit	Interval	Non-Gaussian distribution Mode, median, percentiles Gaussian distribution Mean, standard deviation
Serum glucose concentration	mmol/L	Ratio	Non-Gaussian distribution Mode, median, percentiles Gaussian distribution Mean, standard deviation

A **ratio** scale is the same as an interval scale—that is, a continuous scale with equal-sized intervals—but with an absolute zero point where the property does not exist. Height in centimeters and glucose in mmol/L are examples of ratio scales. The types of statistics that are used to describe data are restricted somewhat by the scale of measurement. The mean, for example, should not be used to describe central tendency for an ordinal measurement.

The scale of measurement for many properties is arbitrary, depending on methods available, convenience, tradition, and other factors. Ratio and interval scales are often preferred because they provide more information and permit more-precise comparisons of measurements at different times and locations, which is helpful for medical and quality assurance decisions.

When a property is measured on a scale, we refer to it as a variable. A **variable** is a **property** of the animal with a **scale of measurement** applied to it. For example, if the property is number of blood neutrophils, the corresponding variable could be neutrophils/L of blood. Each observation or result of a variable is called a **value** (e.g., 11.1×10^9/L). In order to judge the medical meaning of a particular value, we often compare it with the expected value in some **population**. Reference intervals used to interpret laboratory results are examples of expected population values. To obtain the exact population value would require measuring the property in all members of the population. This is not practically feasible, so we take measurements instead on a smaller **sample** of the population and use the sample value to estimate the population value. The accuracy of the population estimate depends on how the sample was obtained and on the size of the sample. Generally, the larger the sample, the better it represents the population; **random** sampling avoids bias in the population estimate.

The set of values for a population or a sample is often summarized by three characteristics: (1) a measure of central tendency (mode, median, or mean), (2) a measure of variation about the center (standard deviation or interpercentile interval), and (3) an indication of the shape of the distribution of values (Gaussian, skewed, multimodal).

Measures of Central Tendency

The **mode** is the most frequently occurring value in a set of values. The **median** is the middle value in a series of ordered values. The **mean** $(\bar{x})$ is the sum of all the individual values divided by the number of values (n):

$$\bar{x} = \frac{\sum x_i}{n}$$

(Equation 3.1)

where x_i represents all the individual values of x, and $\sum$ indicates "the sum of."

Measures of Variation

The **range** is the difference between the smallest and largest value in the data sample. A **percentile** is a specified value that indicates the percentage of values above or below that value. For example, if a calcium concentration of 3.2 mmol/L is the 10.1 percentile, then 10.1% of the calcium values in the sample or population are equal to or below 3.2 mmol/L.

An **interpercentile interval** indicates the upper and lower values within which a certain percentage of the sample or population values occur. For example, the central 95% interval would be bounded by the values that correspond to the 2.5 and the 97.5 percentiles.

The **standard deviation** *(sd)* characterizes the dispersion of values around the mean. It is calculated as the square root of the variance. Of the following two equivalent formulae, the latter is easier for calculating the standard deviation.

$$sd = \sqrt{\frac{\sum(x_i - x)^2}{n-1}} = \sqrt{\sum x_i^2 - \frac{\left(\sum x_i\right)^2}{n}}$$

(Equation 3.2)

For some evaluations of precision of an analytic procedure, it is helpful to have a measure of dispersion in relation to the size of the mean. The **coefficient of** variation (CV) is a measure of variation relative to the mean, in which the standard deviation is divided by the mean and multiplied by 100%.

$$CV = \frac{sd(100\%)}{mean}$$ (Equation 3.3)

A CV allows comparisons of variation between methods. However, the CV is not independent of the concentration. For any particular method, it is not uncommon to find a higher CV in control samples at lower concentrations.

If we measure the same quantity on several random samples of the same population and calculate the mean for each sample, the standard error of the mean can be calculated as a measure of the variation among these means. The standard error of the mean for a population can be estimated from one sample as follows:

$$s_{\bar{x}} = \frac{sd}{\sqrt{n}}$$ (Equation 3.4)

where $s_{\bar{x}}$ represents the standard error of the mean, sd is the standard deviation, and n is the sample size.

Data Distribution

Biological data can appear in many possible distributions. The symmetrical **Gaussian distribution** ("normal" distribution) is most familiar, and several of the commonly used parametric statistics, including mean, sd, t-tests, and F-tests, assume that the population data has a Gaussian distribution. However, data can be distributed in many other ways, including flattened (**kurtosis**), positively or negatively **skewed,** or **multimodal,** as illustrated in Figure 3.1. If the assumption of a Gaussian distribution is not warranted, the data can be described by using the median and percentiles, and inferences can be drawn by using nonparametric methods, which are described in textbooks of statistics. In a Gaussian distribution the mode, median, and mean have the same value, whereas in a non-normal distribution each measure of central tendency can have a different value (Fig. 3.2). In contrast to the mode and the mean, the median describes a true measure of the center for all distributions—half of the values are greater than the median, and half are less than the median.

Confidence Intervals

A **confidence interval** is a range of values around a statistic that has a known probability of containing the true population value. In a Gaussian (normal) distri-

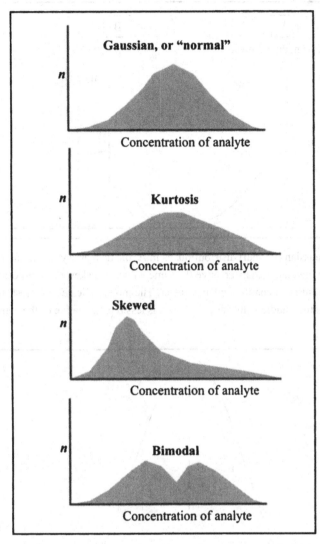

Figure 3.1. Biological data may be distributed in many ways, some of which are illustrated here. Valid statistical descriptions and inferential procedures depend on the type of distribution.

bution, the mean and standard deviation can be used to describe the proportion of values falling within a particular area of the normal curve. As illustrated in Figure 3.3, the area under a perfect Gaussian distribution from -1 *sd* to $+1$ *sd* represents 68% of the values. The area from -2 *sd* to $+2$ *sd* represents 95%, and the area between -3 *sd* and $+3$ *sd* represents 99% of the values. These intervals that contain a certain percentage of the values are termed confidence intervals. If, for example, the mean of a group of normally distributed calcium values is 9.1 mmol/L, and 1 *sd* is 0.2 mmol/L, then you could have 95% confidence that the sample mean lies in the range between the mean $\pm$ 2 *sd,* that is, between 8.7 and 9.5 mmol/L. This would be called the **95% confidence interval.**

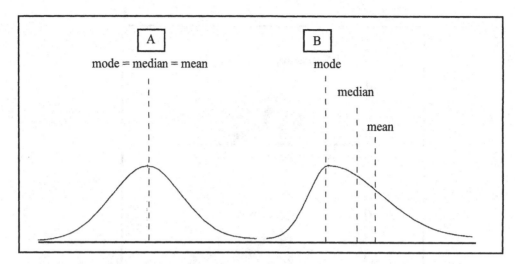

Figure 3.2. In a Gaussian (normal) distribution, as in A, the data are symmetrical about the center and the mode, median, and mean have the same value. In a skewed (non-normal) distribution, as in B, the measures of central tendency differ. The mode indicates the most frequent value, the median indicates the middle value, and the mean is less representative of the center of distribution.

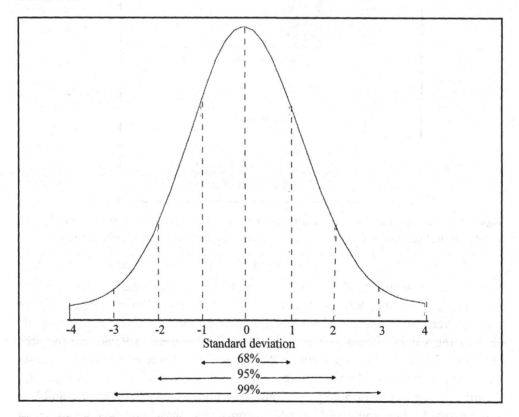

Figure 3.3. In a Gaussian distribution with a mean of 0, the proportion of values in each standard deviation interval can be determined. The intervals that contain a certain percentage of the values are called confidence intervals.

Accuracy, Precision, and Allowable Error

Accuracy and precision are distinctly different concepts (Fig. 3.4). Accuracy describes how well the method obtains the true value. **Accuracy** is a measure of the systematic error between a sample value and the true value. In a group of replicate analyses of a sample, the closer the determined mean comes to the true or known value, the more accurate is the method. **Precision** is the random variation in a set of replicate measurements. Precision describes the reproducibility of the method, or how well replicate measurements of the same sample agree with one another. In a group of replicate analyses of a sample, the smaller the standard deviation (the narrower the distribution), the more precise is the method. In Figure 3.5, method A is more precise (the distribution of values is narrower) but less accurate (the mean is further from the true value) than method B.

Accuracy and precision are important to evaluating and selecting a laboratory procedure as well as to interpreting the test result. As illustrated in Figure 2.1 and discussed in Chapter 2, assessing accuracy (systematic analytic error) and precision (random analytic error) determines the total analytic error of a procedure. For a test result to be useful, the clinician or other user must be able to assume that the total analytic error is less than the allowable error for that result. **Allowable error** is defined as the maximum error allowed in an analytic procedure for its test results to be medically useful. For example, a serum potassium concentration that exceeds 8.0 mmol/L can lead to serious cardiac problems. If the clinician considers that it is important to be able to interpret a reported potassium value of 8.0 mmol/L as somewhere in the range of 7.6 to 8.4 mmol/L, then the allowable error is $\pm 5\%$. For a potassium method to be useful, the total analytic error of the method (systematic plus random) must be less than this allowable error of 5%. If the total analytic error of a procedure exceeds the allowable error, the method will not be useful for valid medical decisions and should not be instituted in the laboratory.

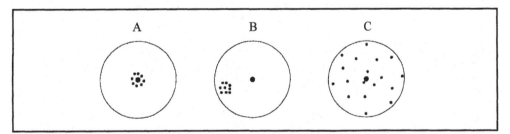

Figure 3.4. The large dot in the center of each target represents the true value for each of three methods (A, B, and C), and the small dots indicate the results of samples run on each method. The results in A indicate that the method is both accurate and precise; the results in B, that it is precise but inaccurate; the results in C, that it is accurate but imprecise.

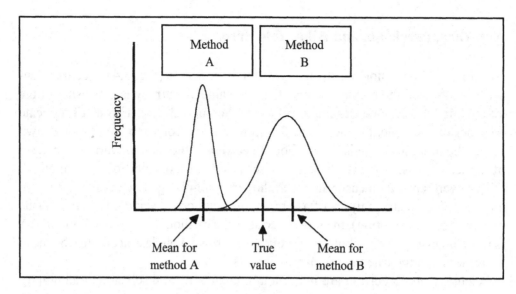

Figure 3.5. Frequency distributions for two methods, A and B. Method A is much more precise than method B, but method B is more accurate than method A.

Chapter 4

Monitoring for Quality

After the laboratory has established its quality goals, a quality control system must be put in place to continuously monitor the analytic procedures, thus ensuring that the quality goals are being met. A quality control system monitors quality at three levels. First, over the short term (daily), the system monitors for systematic and random errors in each run of a procedure to ensure that the patient's sample results are acceptable. Second, the system monitors over the medium term (weeks to months) to ensure that the analytical procedures remain free of significant random errors and slowly developing systematic errors. Third, using accumulated quality control and proficiency testing data, the system monitors the procedures over the long term (months to years) to ensure that they are as accurate and precise as possible. A quality control monitoring system consists of internal quality control measures and external quality assurance testing (proficiency testing).

Internal Monitoring—Quality Control

CONTINUOUS (INTERVAL OR RATIO SCALE) MEASUREMENTS
Most tests in clinical chemistry, and many in hematology and the other disciplines, use interval or ratio scale measurements, allowing the application of the common statistical measures for quality control procedures. Daily quality control of laboratory procedures is essential to detect potential errors that can result from faulty reagents, malfunctioning equipment, or technician error. One, two, or more control materials should be analyzed with each run of unknown samples.

Selecting and Preparing Quality Control Materials. The quality control material should resemble the samples it accompanies in the run. If the samples are serum, the controls should ideally be serum. If the samples are urine, the controls should be urine. Because controls accompany samples in every analytic run, a large volume of control material is required every year. The pool of control material can be commercial lyophilized material or unused patient samples that have

2 5

been pooled and frozen. Frozen liquid pools tend to show slightly less random variation than lyophilized pools, but liquid pools can deteriorate if transported in unsatisfactory conditions. Lyophilized material should be reconstituted carefully, with slow mixing to avoid denaturing the protein. Frozen control material should be mixed gently after thawing, to disperse constituents that have accumulated near the bottom during freezing. Control material prepared from pooled patient samples can contain infectious agents; the pool can be tested for specific agents that are undesirable. Long-term stability is important for control material, so the laboratory requires sufficient freezer and refrigerator space to accommodate 1–2 years' supply. The control material must be stable during storage and available in sufficient quantity in separate vials for periodic analysis over long periods of time (6 months or, preferably, 1 year). New lots of control material should be tested in parallel with the current lot over a 3-week period to ensure consistency of results. Care should be taken to avoid using control material beyond its expiration date. Reconstituted control material usually has a short shelf life (1–2 days, usually; check with the manufacturer where appropriate).

Calculating Control Limits and Target Means. Before a quality control chart can be prepared, target values for the mean and standard deviation of the controls must be calculated. Temporary values for the mean and standard deviation can be determined by running the controls in duplicate for 20 days and using the 40 values for the initial calculations. These temporary target values are used for quality control for 2–3 months while additional control data is collected. The **cumulative mean target value** and the **usual standard deviation** can then be calculated from a series of 3 or 4 monthly values. The usual standard deviation should be equal to or less than the precision goals established for the laboratory (as described in Tables 2.1 and 2.2). **Control limits** are the limits within which control values for a laboratory procedure must be for a patient sample result to be considered valid. The control limits are commonly set at the mean plus or minus either 2, 2.5, or 3 standard deviations, depending on several factors that are discussed below.

Levey-Jennings Control Charts. Two important decisions that must be made regarding a quality control procedure are (1) how many control materials should be used per run of samples (1, 2, 3, or more)? and (2) what control rules should be used as the warning and/or rejection signals to indicate that there is a problem with the test? Before making these decisions, there are several factors to consider, which are discussed in more detail later in this chapter. For now, we will describe the commonly used quality control process in which two control materials accompany each run of samples and there is one rejection rule, the 1_{2s} control rule, which indicates that if either one of the control values exceeds the mean plus or minus 2 standard deviations, the run should be rejected (Fig. 4.1).

The control charts for this one-rule system could be prepared as in Figure 4.1.

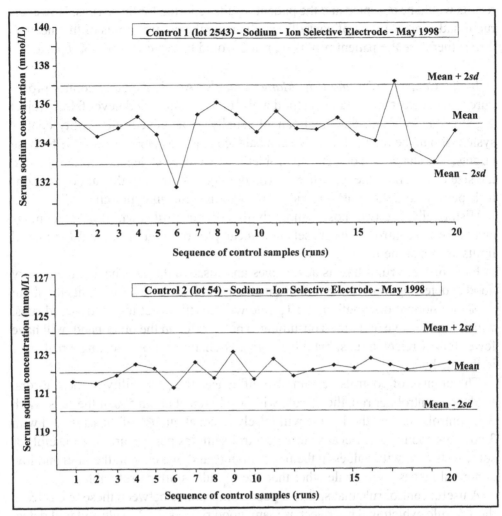

Figure 4.1. Example of a Levey-Jennings control chart for internal quality control of the procedure to measure serum sodium concentration. According to the 1_{2s} control rule described in the text, two runs (6 and 17) would be rejected because control 1 was outside the target range of the mean $\pm$ 2 *sd.*

Time (labeled as days or runs) is on the *x*-axis, and the measured variable with the appropriate units (serum sodium concentration in the example) is labeled on the *y*-axis. A scale on the *y*-axis set to accommodate a change of 4 or 5 standard deviations from the mean in the control value is usually sufficient. It is also useful to print on the chart the time period over which the chart was used and the instrument or analytical method used. The target values—the expected mean and the control limits at the mean +2 *sd* and the mean −2 *sd*—are then drawn on the chart as easily visible horizontal lines. Next, individual control sample values are plotted sequentially on the chart to determine whether they are "in control" or "out of control." In the example illustrated in Figure 4.1, according to the 1_{2s} rule described above, both of the control values for runs 1, 2, 3, 4, and 5 were "in control"; therefore the results would be accepted and the patient results reported for those runs. However, run 6 had control 1 "out of control" (i.e., outside the control limits of the mean $\pm$ 2 sd); therefore the patient results on run 6 would be rejected and not reported.

Which Control Rules and How Many Controls? An ideal quality control procedure would detect an unstable method with 100% certainty and never falsely reject a good run. Although this ideal cannot usually be achieved, the quality control system should be planned to arrive at a balance that is as close as possible to these targets. The chances of detecting a problem with a method depend on four factors: the size of the error, the type of error (random or systematic), the number of controls per run, and the control rules used to evaluate the analytic run.

Historically, the two most commonly used control rules with Levey-Jennings charts are **1_{2s}** (control limits are set at the mean plus or minus 2 sd) and **1_{3s}** (control limits are set at the mean $\pm$ 3 sd).

Each of these rules has its advantages and disadvantages. The 1_{2s} rule is very good at detecting most real errors in a method, but because 2 sd accounts for about 95% of a normal distribution, the 1_{2s} rule will falsely reject too many good runs, which is expensive and time-consuming. The 1_{3s} rule, on the other hand, will have fewer falsely rejected runs, but it has a greater chance of not detecting a real error in the method.

The number of controls per run also influences the probability of these errors. With one control per run, the 1_{2s} rule will falsely reject about 5% of the runs. With two controls per run, the 1_{2s} rule will falsely reject about 9% of the runs, and with 3 controls about 14%. Because three control samples per run are often useful for some tests (one with values in the normal range and one each in the high and low abnormal ranges), some rule other than the 1_{2s} rule is often preferable.

A useful control rule that strikes a good compromise between these two rules is the **$1_{2.5s}$** rule, which will not reject as many good runs as the 1_{2s} rule and will detect more of the real errors than the 1_{3s} rule.

Another factor to consider is that an effective quality control procedure should detect both systematic and random errors in a method. Each of the various rules recommended for quality control is better at detecting one or the other of these error types. Random errors, which suggest a precision problem with the method, show up on control charts as an increase in the distribution width of control values. Systematic errors, which suggest an accuracy problem, show up on control charts as a series of control values moving in one direction, often remaining on one side of the mean, for example. The $1_{2.5s}$ rule therefore is good at detecting random errors but will not be as effective for systematic errors unless they are large.

To detect both random and systematic errors more effectively, multiple-rule quality control procedures like those proposed by Westgard can be used. A control chart advocated by Westgard for chemistry analyses includes a **cumulative mean value** (calculated initially after 20 measurements have been done) and a series of control limits drawn at the $\pm$ **1** *sd;* the **mean** $\pm$ **2** *sd;* the **mean** $\pm$ **3** *sd;* and the **mean** $\pm$ **4** *sd,* as illustrated in Figure 4.2.

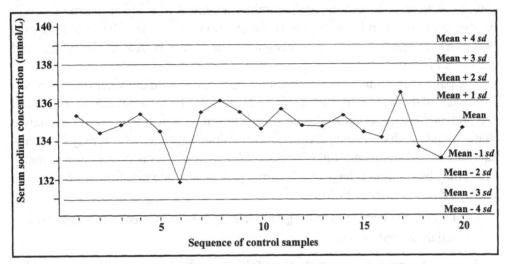

Figure 4.2. Example of a Westgard control chart for internal monitoring of laboratory results for errors. Control values falling outside acceptable limits or control values repeatedly following a trend are warnings to laboratory personnel that corrective action is necessary.

As with the Levey-Jennings chart, the control values are plotted sequentially on the chart. Changes in these values are then used to assess the quality of the results using a set of several rules. The following Westgard Multi-Rule Procedure[9] is an example of one multiple rule procedure used to control for both random and systematic errors in a chemistry laboratory. In this procedure, a control value is **in control** unless one or more of the following rules are violated:

- **1₂ₛ, 1 control value exceeding the mean** $\pm$ **2** *sd*—a warning rule to initiate further testing of control data by other control rules

- **1₃ₛ, 1 control value exceeding the mean** $\pm$ **3** *sd*—a rejection rule sensitive mainly to random error

- **2₂ₛ, two consecutive control values exceeding the same limit of mean + 2** *sd* **or mean** – **2** *sd*—a rejection rule sensitive to systematic error

- **R₄ₛ, 1 control value exceeding the limit of mean + 2** *sd* **and another exceeding the limit of mean** – **2** *sd*—a rejection rule sensitive to random error

- **4₁ₛ, 4 consecutive control values exceeding the same limit of mean + 1** *sd* **or mean** – **1** *sd*—a rejection rule sensitive to systematic error

- **10ₘₑₐₙ, 10 consecutive control values falling on one side of the mean**—a rejection rule sensitive to systematic error

What is a practical way to select the number of controls per run and the control rules? As the number of controls per run increases, the probability of falsely rejecting a good run increases, but the method must be controlled to ensure that faulty runs are detected. Therefore, use the minimum number of controls per run that will adequately detect a truly faulty run. If, for example, it is known that a method may deteriorate a little over time, controls may be necessary both at the beginning and the end of the run.

The particular control rules adopted for each test should consider the test precision goals of the laboratory (see Tables 2.1 and 2.2), the relative stability of the test method, and the importance of precision at different concentrations of the analyte that coincide with critical medical decision points. In some cases it may be necessary to have a complex multiple rule procedure as described above. For other methods it may be suitable to have two controls per run and one rule for each of random and systematic errors as follows:

- $1_{2.5s}$, **1 control value exceeding the mean $\pm$ 2.5 *sd*—**a rejection rule sensitive mainly to random error

- 8_{mean}, **8 consecutive control values falling on one side of the mean—**a rejection rule sensitive to systematic error

Errors and Corrective Actions for Rejection Rules. Based on the control rule(s) violated and the number of controls per run, examine the procedure for the likely error.

Systematic errors often result from instrument or calibration problems. Check for improperly functioning instruments (e.g., a pipette that is dispensing slightly less or slightly more of a reagent). Check for contaminated, unstable, or improperly prepared standards or calibrators or a nonlinear calibration curve.

Random errors often result from instability in instruments, resulting in random changes in temperature or timing of a procedure, or from inconsistencies in the manner in which technologists prepare, mix, or pipette samples or reagents

When analytic control problems occur, they can often be resolved using a step-by-step procedure that looks at the common and simpler causes first, followed by the more complex difficulties. Each of the following steps can be tried in turn to resolve the problems.

1. Check for the most obvious problems, such as reagent depletion, mechanical faults, or clots, and if such problems are found, repeat the control assays.

2. Use another aliquot of control material and repeat the control assays.

3. Use freshly reconstituted control material and repeat the control assays.

4. Use a new lot of reagent(s), recalibrate equipment, and repeat the control assays.

5. Run routine instrument maintenance, recalibrate equipment, and repeat the control assays.

6. Consult the manufacturer if appropriate, follow suggestions, and repeat the control assays.

If one of the above or similar steps results in acceptable control values, repeat the run of samples on the disputed run, and if the controls are acceptable, report the patient test results. If it is not possible to correct the control problem quickly, it may be necessary to suspend the procedure until the problem is corrected. All staff should be notified of the suspended procedure, and no patient test results should be reported from the out-of-control run. The test can be done by an alternative method, if available, or the sample may be sent to another laboratory. In either case the clinician ordering the test should be informed of the problem and of any delays that might occur. Every quality control decision should be recorded in the laboratory quality manual. Control problems should be recorded with time and date, method, analyte, description of the problem, how the problem was corrected, staff involved, and actions taken with patient samples.

Calibrators, Controls, Reagents, and Instruments. Calibrators and controls serve different functions. **Calibrators** have values established by the manufacturer (using definitive or reference methods) that are used to correlate the output of an instrument with a known concentration of analyte. Calibrators are used to set the reported values for an analyte accurately. **Controls** are used to check both on the accuracy of the calibration and on the stability of the instrument and other aspects of the method. Calibrators should be purchased in lots large enough to last a year or more to ensure stability. A new lot of calibrators should be tested for some time with the previous lot to ensure consistency. Reagents and instruments should also be checked for quality. New lots of reagent can be assumed acceptable if on their use the controls are on target (in control). Similarly, controls tested on an instrument after maintenance will determine the acceptability of instrument performance.

When a new instrument or reagent testing system is being selected for a laboratory, the laboratory should ask the manufacturer for the performance specifications. Prior to purchase, the new instrument and/or reagent systems should be tested to ensure that these performance specifications are met in the laboratory and that they meet the quality goals of the laboratory.

Definitive and Reference Methods and Reference Materials. The National Reference System for the Clinical Laboratory (NRSCL) of the United States has established a number of definitive and reference methods for many of the analytes of interest to diagnostic laboratories. **Definitive methods** are the most accurate. They usually purify the analyte of concern by a separation procedure and measure its concentration on the most accurate, precise, and sensitive instruments available. These methods are available in the United States in the National Institute of Standards and Technology, in the Centers for Disease Control and Prevention, and in some other large laboratories. **Reference methods** are slightly less rigorously standardized than definitive methods, but their accuracy has been repeatedly tested and found to be very good. Many large hospital laboratories use reference methods. **Reference materials** are commercially available materials that may be used as controls or calibrators. The true concentrations of analytes in these materials has been set using definitive or reference methods.

CATEGORICAL (NOMINAL SCALE) MEASUREMENTS
Internal quality control methods to detect potential reagent, equipment, or human errors for procedures with mainly categorical results (e.g., cytopathology, histopathology, microbiology, and some aspects of hematology) consist of using standards and controls where applicable, stepwise inspection protocols, and periodic internal audits of the procedures.

Controls and Inspections. In microbiological laboratories, samples of new media should be checked for sterility by incubating without added bacteria. Media and reagents, whether produced locally or purchased from a commercial supplier, should be checked regularly with internal control or stock organisms to verify that the reagents produce the true positive or negative reactions expected in the various test procedures. Similarly, antibiotic sensitivity control testing can be done with known organisms of known sensitivity to ensure that the procedure is working accurately. Sources of problems are usually detected by stepwise inspections of the procedure.

In a histopathology laboratory, specimens are collected, transported, fixed, processed, stained, mounted on slides, described and evaluated by a pathologist, and reported. Errors can occur in one or more of these steps and potentially compromise the accuracy of the final report. Control blocks of tissue can be cut, stained, and mounted along with each set of patient specimens to control for errors in these procedures. The control samples are examined at the end of each run for section thickness, microtome marks, and staining characteristics to ensure consistency with those of previously processed controls. Examining stained material to detect microorganisms or specific tissue or cell components depends on consistent and often subtle differences in staining characteristics of the various components of the preparation. Stains can deteriorate, be improperly prepared, or be affected by other aspects of specimen collection and processing. New batches of stain should be checked for accuracy by using a standard tissue or microorganism preparation of known composition. Control material for specific components (e.g., amyloid, Gram-positive bacteria) can be prepared in-house or purchased from commercial suppliers. Problems encountered are usually solved by stepwise inspection of the procedure.

Internal Audits for Quality Assessment. Another approach to evaluating the quality of categorical laboratory procedures is the internal audit. A random sample of previous cases is selected and evaluated for quality once or twice each year. Individuals, using audit forms prepared for the specific discipline, apply a grade to certain aspects of the procedure that are considered important to the quality of the result. The results are summarized, and the ranked scores can be analyzed to show differences from one audit to the next. Processes requiring attention become apparent. The aspects of the procedure addressed in the audit, the sample size, and the frequency of audits depend on the time and finances available and the desired confidence in the results. A minimum sample size of 50 and a minimum frequency of one audit per year are recommended. Examples of internal audit forms for histopathology, cytopathology, and blood smear evaluation in hematology are illustrated in Figures 4.3 and 4.4.

External Monitoring—Proficiency Testing

External quality assurance programs, which are standard practice in human health laboratories, should also be an essential part of the quality control procedures in veterinary laboratories. External quality assurance programs provide laboratories with an unbiased external measure of the accuracy of their procedures. For laboratory procedures whose results are measured on continuous interval scales (e.g., clinical chemistry, hematology, endocrinology, serology, therapeutic drug monitoring), external quality assurance procedures can detect slowly developing systematic errors that may be missed with internal quality control procedures. External quality assurance programs are especially important for laboratory procedures that provide discrete categorical results (cytopathology, histopathology, bacteriology, parasitology, and some aspects of hematology). The external quality assurance program sometimes provides the only objective check on the accuracy of the categorical results.

External quality assurance programs provide each participating laboratory with an aliquot or replicate of the same specimen and ask each laboratory to analyze the material for one or more variables. The results of the participating laboratories are returned for data analysis to the agency sponsoring the external program. Reports summarizing the results are distributed to the participating laboratories usually 3–4 weeks after submission. The reports consist of statistical summaries and plots indicating how the results of the participating laboratory compare with the results of the peer group. In most external assessments the true value, or benchmark, for each analysis is considered to be the mean (or median or mode) value of the group. In others, the benchmark may be the value obtained by a standard reference method or the mean of a group of reference laboratories (these are less favorable because of the small sample size).

Internal Audit Form – Histopathology

Case Number: _____

Species: _____ Breed: _____ Age: _____ Sex: _____

Submission Date/Time: _____

Report Date/Time: _____

Turnover Time: _____

Gross Path Description:	☐ Good,	☐ Adequate,	☐ Minor error,	☐ Major error,	☐ NA
Specimen Quality:	☐ Good,	☐ Adequate,	☐ Minor error,	☐ Major error,	☐ NA
Section Quality:	☐ Good,	☐ Adequate,	☐ Minor error,	☐ Major error,	☐ NA
Stain Quality:	☐ Good,	☐ Adequate,	☐ Minor error,	☐ Major error,	☐ NA
Histopathologic description:	☐ Good,	☐ Adequate,	☐ Minor error,	☐ Major error,	☐ NA

Special stains requested: ☐ Yes ☐ No
Special stains required: ☐ Yes ☐ No

Original Diagnosis: _____

Audit Diagnosis: _____

Comments: _____

_____

Recommended Actions: _____

Internal Audit Form – Cytopathology

Case Number: _____

Species: _____ Breed: _____ Age: _____ Sex: _____

Submission Date/Time: _____

Report Date/Time: _____

Turnover Time: _____

Specimen Quality:	☐ Good,	☐ Adequate,	☐ Minor error,	☐ Major error,	☐ NA
Smear Quality:	☐ Good,	☐ Adequate,	☐ Minor error,	☐ Major error,	☐ NA
Stain Quality:	☐ Good,	☐ Adequate,	☐ Minor error,	☐ Major error,	☐ NA
Cytopathologic description:	☐ Good,	☐ Adequate,	☐ Minor error,	☐ Major error,	☐ NA

Special stains requested: ☐ Yes ☐ No
Special stains required: ☐ Yes ☐ No

Original Diagnosis: _____

Audit Diagnosis: _____

Comments: _____

_____

Recommended Actions: _____

Figure 4.3. Examples of internal audit forms for evaluating quality of histopathological and cytopathological procedures.

Internal Audit Form – Blood Smear Evaluation

Case Number: _____

Species: _____ Breed: _____ Age: _____ Sex: _____

Receipt Date/Time:_____ Report Date:/Time: _____ Turnaround Time: _____

CHARACTERISTICS (Units)	ORIGINAL RESULT	AUDIT RESULT
Smear quality (0 to ++++)		
Stain quality (0 to ++++)		
Total WBC ($\times 10^9$/L)		
Segmented neutrophils (%)		
Band neutrophils (%)		
Metamyelocytes (%)		
Eosinophils (%)		
Basophils (%)		
Lymphocytes (%)		
Monocytes (%)		
Disintegrated cells (%)		
Reticulocytes (%)		
Immature lymphocytes (yes/no)		
Heinz bodies (0 to ++++)		
Polychromasia (0 to ++++)		
Anisocytosis (0 to ++++)		
Microcytosis (0 to ++++)		
Macrocytosis (0 to ++++)		
Hypochromasia (0 to ++++)		
Poikilocytosis (0 to ++++)		
Crenation/burr cells (0 to ++++)		
Leptocytes (0 to ++++)		
Basophilic stippling (0 to ++++)		
Toxic granulation (0 to ++++)		
Mast cells (yes/no)		
Hemobartonella (yes/no)		
Pathologist's interpretation		

Auditor's Comments: _____

Recommended Actions:_____

Figure 4.4. Example of an internal audit form for quality assessment of blood smear evaluation.

An example of an external quality assurance program for veterinary laboratories is the Veterinary Laboratory Association Quality Assurance Program® (VLAQAP). The program consists of eight sample modules that are offered four times each year to each participating laboratory. The modules cover the following disciplines: chemistry, endocrinology, serology, parasitology, hematology, therapeutic drug monitoring, bacteriology, and histopathology. Each laboratory can select which of the modules meets its needs. The standard eight modules contain material from a dog, a cat, or a horse. Also, one additional hematology and chemistry module is available for other species (e.g., cow, sheep, pig, rodent, fish, avian) if desired. Each participant receives graphical reports each quarter, showing its results and how they relate to the group results. The results are categorized by method and/or instrument when appropriate. In addition, the program offers detailed descriptive reports by a pathologist or microbiologist on the categorical results for hematology, bacteriology, parasitology, and histopathology. Figure 4.5 illustrates the type of feedback information received from external quality assurance programs.

External quality assurance programs indicate not only which procedures are inaccurate and require attention but also which procedures are performing well in other laboratories and may be worth considering for introduction into your laboratory.

In the example in Figure 4.5, the participant's sodium result of 159.2 mmol/L is 3 units from the group mean, yet it is still within the mean plus or minus 2 *sd* of the group. This result would not likely require any action, but if in the subsequent external test, the sodium was further from the mean in the same direction (e.g., 162 mmol/L), the laboratory would have reason to examine the procedure.

The breakdown by instrument/method provides the laboratory with information about other methods that are available for the procedure and the precision that other laboratories are getting with alternate methods. The value of an external quality assurance program is proportional to the number of participants. The mean values and measures of precision are valuable as benchmarks for accuracy if there are sufficiently large numbers of laboratories in the group.

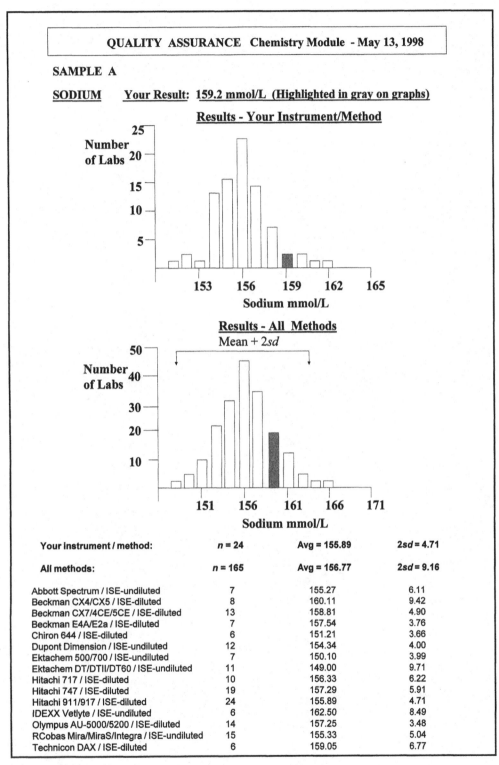

Figure 4.5. Example of types of information available from an external quality assurance program.

Chapter 5

Quality of Operations, Policies, and Resources

Mandate, Services, Clients, Organizational Structure, and Budget

For the laboratory quality manual, the description of the laboratory should summarize the mandate and mission, the types of services offered, the intended clients, and the budget. The mandate and mission describe the service goals and expectations for the laboratory, which can influence the types of quality assurance procedures considered and the methods of incorporating costs associated with quality assurance. For example, a commercial diagnostic laboratory may function totally for clients who request service on a fee-for-service basis. The quality assurance costs would usually be incorporated into the fees for the various test procedures. Alternatively, a state or provincial government laboratory may be mandated to do specific testing for the agricultural community with a specific budget supplied for that service. Costs associated with quality assurance may be allocated to a specific quality assurance budget in such circumstances. A laboratory affiliated with a veterinary college may do similar diagnostic testing on a fee-for-service basis, but it may also be mandated to play an educational or research role for the veterinary college. Additional testing, which could be helpful for student training but not essential in a routine diagnostic setting, may require different considerations for quality assurance and cost allocation.

The various services offered by the laboratory should be listed in the laboratory quality manual. The scope and diversity of laboratory activities are important determinants of the types of quality assurance procedures that are likely to be helpful. For example, a large laboratory doing chemistry, hematology, endocrinology, microbiology, cytology, histopathology, and parasitology in different subsections of a large building may be able to improve its quality assurance by developing an electronic system that keeps track of every specimen and its stage of analysis. A small laboratory doing two or three specialized assays is less likely to find such a system cost-effective.

The intended clients served by the laboratory are also an important consideration for quality issues. Practicing veterinarians may wish to have laboratory results reported with specific types of reference ranges, whereas clients doing research studies may be more interested in results reported with the test characteristics (precision and accuracy) of a given procedure. Frequent client consultation, by questionnaire or other means, is essential to developing and improving a laboratory quality assurance system.

The organizational structure of the laboratory should clearly indicate the individual(s) responsible for the various laboratory activities, including who is responsible for each aspect of the quality assurance program. Some large laboratories have a director or manager of quality assurance. Individuals in the laboratory may be assigned specific quality assurance tasks, or a quality assurance committee may be part of the structure. Problem-solving teams may be assembled for troubleshooting with specific automated instruments. These types of quality assurance-related individuals or groups should be described or illustrated in a flow chart in this section of the manual.

The budget information in the laboratory quality manual, for the most part, can be a summary but with details on the quality assurance budget items. The individual(s) with responsibility and authority for expenditures on quality assurance items should be indicated.

Policies, Procedures, and Laboratory Management

Commitment to quality by all personnel is essential to an effective quality assurance program. Ensuring quality requires attention to every laboratory activity and must therefore involve the director, supervisors, analysts, and clerical staff. The personnel of the laboratory should be described in the manual, with a listing of their education, experience, and continuing education and professional development activities. Laboratories with competent and experienced personnel who have frequently attended continuing education courses in quality assurance and laboratory methods show a commitment to quality.

Hiring policies and procedures should result in well-qualified, certified technologists who have training in quality assurance practices as well as in laboratory methods. The interview process for new staff should determine their knowledge of quality assurance concepts and procedures. Each laboratory should have at least one individual who is sufficiently knowledgeable about quality assurance not only to oversee quality in the laboratory but also to provide periodic in-house quality assurance workshops to the staff. The laboratory director or manager is ideal for this role; when budget decisions are made by the individual(s) responsible for quality assurance, the costs for quality are considered with those of other aspects of laboratory activity.

Each laboratory should have a standard orientation and training program for new employees. Each new employee should be thoroughly trained in the methods they will use. New staff should be oriented to the laboratory's quality assurance program, to the equipment they will operate, and to the safety procedures of the laboratory.

Continuing education and feedback on performance are also important. An effective means of promoting quality in the operations of the laboratory is to make available to personnel regular professional development programs for improving their knowledge and competence. Similarly, periodic quality assurance workshops for staff reinforce the value of and the procedures necessary for ensuring quality results. Performance assessments of personnel should be regular and include an evaluation of their role in the quality assurance program.

To help everyone understand the chain of authority and how information flows, the laboratory should have an organizational chart showing the direct and courtesy reporting relationships among members of the laboratory, as well as the lines of reporting to people outside the laboratory.

Diagnostic laboratories are often subdivided into sections or units that are based historically on discipline specialties. Although this basis of subdivision may be appropriate, it may be more advantageous to subdivide the diagnostic laboratory into sections or units aimed at the most efficient and flexible use of resources (space, personnel, equipment, and supplies) in order to meet the diagnostic service demands more cost-effectively.

The education, certification, and experience of the laboratory director and laboratory manager are especially important to how well the diagnostic laboratory achieves its goals. The laboratory director should be a licensed DVM with a graduate degree and/or board certification in an appropriate discipline and at least 2 years of experience supervising laboratory testing. The laboratory manager should have a bachelor's or master's degree in medical technology or one of the biological or chemical sciences, a minimum of 2 years of laboratory training/certification, and 2–3 years of supervisory laboratory experience.

The laboratory manager must be an effective communicator with both the clients and the personnel of the laboratory. The clients must be constantly informed of the laboratory's progress in achieving its goals (e.g., new tests, new methods, tests available, changes in sample requirements or reference ranges). The laboratory manager must also remain in constant communication with the laboratory staff. Regular meetings are an important means of staying in touch and solving problems in their early stages. Minutes should be taken at the meetings and should clearly state the outcome. Problems addressed should be documented by stating the problem and describing the action plan. The problems should be reevaluated at subsequent meetings to determine if they have been corrected and, if not, what additional action may be necessary. The staff must remain motivated to achieve the laboratory's goals through positive and sometimes negative two-way feedback. The laboratory staff must be involved with planning, setting objectives, and problem solving to meet the laboratory goals. To do this the staff must have a clear understanding of the workload necessary to meet the service demands, the resources available, and the long-term goals of the laboratory. A laboratory manager who involves the staff in these activities will gain their trust and respect. Careful attention to the work capacity of the staff is important; the number of personnel must be adequate to the workload to avoid frustration, burnout, and problems with the quality of service. Laboratory staffing must account for vacation leave, sick leave, and personal leave. Each laboratory position must be staffed with from 1.3 to 2.0 individuals, depending on the hours of service coverage required each week by the laboratory. Attention to the relative abilities of technologists may also be necessary to balance strengths and weaknesses when planning work schedules.

The laboratory director or manager should identify any needs for in-service training for the types of work required of specific staff. In addition, any remedial training or continuing education to improve skills should be identified. The laboratory director or manager should maintain a current list of local, regional, and national continuing education programs and meetings that meet the needs of laboratory personnel and should encourage their attendance. Attendance at continuing education programs by staff should be documented and recorded in each employee's personnel file and in the laboratory quality manual.

The laboratory manager is responsible for managing the laboratory's resources, including staff, supplies, and equipment, to provide the services expected. The services expected (range of tests, frequency of testing, cost of tests, turnaround time) are developed through ongoing discussions with users to determine their needs. To achieve the goals of the laboratory, the laboratory manager should motivate the staff to be innovative by involving them in the planning of laboratory activities to develop cost-effective procedures for providing results of the highest standards. A cooperative group effort in this direction is the most effective way to meet the goals of the laboratory.

Laboratory and Equipment

The laboratory quality manual should contain a description of the laboratory and its equipment, records of laboratory and instrument cleaning schedules, records of equipment function and maintenance checks, and troubleshooting protocols for major analytic instruments.

For optimal analytic work, the laboratory should be clean, well lighted, and uncluttered. Work surfaces should be cleaned regularly after use, to avoid the possibility of sample contamination and to preserve the safety of personnel. Work areas should be organized for the most efficient use of personnel, equipment, and supplies. Procedures done with automated analytic instruments are usually more precise than manual procedures, provided that the instruments have been calibrated correctly, controls are used with each run, and instruments are functioning properly. Analytic instruments should be cleaned daily after use and should have regular function and maintenance checks. Maintenance records should be kept for all instruments to help with troubleshooting when problems arise. Service contracts for heavily used major laboratory equipment should be considered in order to ensure that the instruments are operating adequately at all times. Faulty equipment should be repaired or replaced. An analytic error that results from an equipment problem can arise during one or more of many steps in the analysis. It is therefore essential that at least one technologist in the laboratory be completely familiar with the principles and components of each analytic instrument in order to quickly identify equipment problems that have occurred. Individuals or teams can be assigned to each of the large analytic instruments for problem solving, and a stepwise troubleshooting protocol can be developed to quickly investigate the likely sources of error and the action necessary to correct the problem.

Financial Management

The financial management of a laboratory is extremely important to the quality of its services. Cost accounting methods are becoming essential in most laboratories. Laboratories that operate partially or completely on a fee-for-service basis must use a cost accounting approach in their financial operations. Commercial laboratories are well versed in these methods, but many institutional laboratories now must also adopt cost accounting procedures. As government funding is reduced or phased out, many institutional diagnostic laboratories are expected to become partially or completely self-supporting. In some cases, diagnostic laboratories are being viewed as sources of revenue to replace funds lost in grants to the parent institution. Simplistic approaches to this short-term need for funds can quickly erode the resources of a good laboratory, with an accompanying reduction in the quality of its services.

Institutional laboratories that have been funded with grants for many years have accounting systems that are primarily focused on tracking expenditures; their administrative structures often have little experience with the financial and operational methods necessary to generate revenue in a sustainable manner. Maintaining a viable high-quality laboratory that is also profitable requires methods and attitudes different from those required in a grant-funded laboratory.

Many aspects of financial management are important to quality assurance for a laboratory, but two activities are especially so: (1) strategic investments in key laboratory resources, and (2) a cost accounting approach to budgeting. The laboratory manager should prepare the laboratory's budget (with section heads participating where it is appropriate) and should ensure that the laboratory operates within its budget. When budgets are prepared with expectations for higher profits from increases in test volumes, the resources necessary to generate these profits must also be entered into the budget. As the service demands increase, the operating expenses also increase. For example, if the revenue side of the budget is expected to rise by $100,000 next year because of increases in test volumes, the expenditure side of the budget must also rise proportionately. Cost accounting calculations will indicate what these increased expenditures should be—perhaps $35,000 for additional personnel, $15,000 for additional supplies, and $10,000 for additional equipment to meet the increased service demands. As the caseload increases, more personnel, more reagents, more supplies, and more equipment will be required. Laboratories used as revenue sources without proper attention to cost increases will slowly see their resource base eroded and their staff overloaded to accommodate the inevitable increase in operating requirements.

Cost accounting is a method whereby every cost associated with each item or service offered is identified so that it may be budgeted accurately and recovered in the fee. If financial constraints are pressing, the **cost per test** may also be an important criterion in deciding which of two methods to adopt in a method comparison study. For a diagnostic laboratory, the most important cost accounting activity is calculating the cost of each billable test. The main direct costs considered in the cost-per-test calculation include consumable costs (reagents and supplies), depreciated capital costs, service and repair costs, communication costs, and labor costs. Labor cost is by far the largest component of a test cost, ranging from 75% to more than 85% of the total cost per test. Table 5.1 summarizes the main features of a cost-per-test calculation.

Table 5.1. Example calculation of the direct costs associated with a test

Item Cost	Calculation	Cost per Test ($)
Equipment, $10,000	$10,000 ÷ 5 yr ÷ 6,000 tests	0.33
Consumables, $900	$900 ÷ 6,000 tests	0.15
Service/repair, $1,000	$1,000 ÷ 6,000 tests	0.20
Communications, $500	$500 ÷ 6,000 tests	0.08
Labor and benefits, $24/hr	[(12,000 analyses ÷ 13/hr[a]) × $24/hr] ÷ 6,000 tests	3.69
Total direct cost per test		4.45

[a] The calculations are based on 6,000 patient samples for this test each year which, would result in approximately 12,000 tests per year, considering controls, repeats, dilutions, etc., and expecting this test to be performed and analyzed at 13 tests per hour.

Causes and Control of Preanalytic Variation

Many nonanalytic factors can change the concentrations of one or more analytes in a specimen, so that the laboratory results do not accurately reflect the values in the patient. Developing standard procedures for handling reagents and supplies, as well as for specimen collection, specimen transport, and specimen preservation, can minimize the common sources of preanalytic errors.

HANDLING OF REAGENTS AND SUPPLIES

New analytic reagents, whether purchased or prepared in-house, should be labeled, dated, and tested for effectiveness prior to routine use. A sufficient inventory of supplies should be maintained to allow for delayed or faulty shipments. Consistently accurate procedures require stable materials. Large inventories of certain materials from the same lot can help ensure stability. For other materials with a shorter shelf life, standing orders serve to ensure a steady supply. Lyophilized reagents are usually quite stable but should be dated after reconstitution; reagents prepared in-house should be similarly dated. Any reagents that have reached their expiration date should be discarded. Commercial lyophilized reagents can be made in large lots and are tested by the manufacturer for quality. These reagents from the same lot can be expected to be more stable but should be tested before use. Reagents prepared in-house are usually made in smaller lots, and each lot must be tested for accuracy. Storage conditions for analytic materials vary; the manufacturers' recommendations should be followed carefully.

Standards—that is, materials of known composition—are key components for ensuring accuracy in a quality assurance program. Procedures are often calibrated (or standardized) with one or more standards to give the known result when the standard is analyzed. The accuracy of a procedure is often assessed by determining whether or not the procedure gives the correct result on reference standards of known composition. Chemicals of certified purity and other standard materials are available from commercial companies. Standard reference materials for clinical laboratories are available from the National Bureau of Standards. The main supplier of microbiological standards is the American Type Culture Collection (ATCC).

The types of specimen containers, reaction vessels, storage containers, tubing materials, and cleansing solutions used affect many procedures. Several types of glassware and plasticware are available, but some procedures are affected by components of one type of glass or plastic more than another. These special considerations should be noted for each procedure and recorded in the standard laboratory procedures section of the laboratory quality manual (see "Standard Analytic Procedures," below).

HANDLING OF SPECIMENS

Random and Cyclic Biological Variations. Unpredictable day-to-day changes occur in the concentrations of body constituents in the same individual. This **random biological variation** can be quite small for things like plasma electrolytes but much greater for enzymes, cells, and some hormones. Biological variation cannot be controlled, but it must be taken into account when interpreting changes in laboratory results. Most of the random biological variation will be accounted for in the reference intervals for the various species used to interpret laboratory values.

There are **cyclic variations** in many biological functions that lead to similar cyclic variations in the concentrations of many body constituents. Daily, weekly, or monthly variations occur, for example, with the production of many hormones, the production rates of some cells, the excretion rates of certain electrolytes, and the metabolism of certain drugs. As a result, the concentrations of these constituents in blood or urine fluctuate within certain limits.

Diet-, Stress-, and Exercise-Induced Variation. Food ingestion, dietary changes, stress, and exercise can result in changes in measured variables. After a meal, for example, the concentrations of glucose, insulin, and triglycerides may increase. Stress, by inducing the production of cortisol and catecholamines, can result in sometimes dramatic changes in the concentrations of certain constituents, such as white blood cells and glucose. Muscular exertion will lead to some elevations in muscle enzymes, and rigorous exercise can alter not only enzyme levels but electrolyte and glucose concentrations as well.

Ways to help minimize the chances of interpretive errors due to diet-, stress-, or exercise-induced changes include the following:

1. Obtain a good patient history to determine if rigorous muscle activity or food ingestion has been recent.

2. Specimens for tests affected by food ingestion can be taken after the animal has fasted for some time.

3. If the goal is to detect small changes—in hormone concentrations, for example— it may be preferable to sample at the same time each day to avoid the possible effects of cyclic fluctuations.

4. Although stress is difficult to control, every effort to reduce unnecessary stress during sample collection may be helpful for tests known to be affected by cortisol or catecholamine release.

Variations from Technique of Specimen Collection. Proper preparation of the patient can be important to meaningful results. Some microbiological tests require thorough cleansing and disinfection of the specimen collection site, whereas others do not. The proper specimen is important. For example, venous and arterial blood samples differ in a number of characteristics; venous blood has lower concentrations of oxygen and glucose and higher concentrations of ammonia, carbon dioxide, and organic acids. The preservatives and anticoagulants that are commonly used for blood, urine, or other specimens must also be used with attention to their effects on certain analytes. After blood is removed from the animal and allowed to clot, it separates into a solid component containing cells and fibrin and a liquid component called serum. If an anticoagulant is added prior to collection, the liquid component after centrifugation is called plasma. Although serum and plasma are similar in many respects and can be used for many of the same analyses, there are some differences that must be kept in mind. Plasma differs from serum in that it contains fibrinogen; therefore, the total serum protein concentration of plasma will be from 0.2 to 1.0 g/L higher than that of serum, depending on the species and the presence of inflammation. Clotting also releases potassium from platelets, which can slightly increase the potassium concentration of serum.

To avoid waiting for clotting, heparinized plasma is often used when blood chemistry analyses are required quickly. Sometimes in these circumstances, as well as when insufficient clotting time is allowed for serum collection, small fibrin clots can form in the separated sample and lead to problems in the analytic system (e.g., plugging probes or tubes) and cause either erroneous results or instrument problems.

Sometimes blood samples collected for serum analysis can become contaminated with EDTA (ethylenediaminetetraacetic acid), resulting in erroneous values. EDTA chelates cations like iron, magnesium, and calcium, thereby falsely reducing not only the values of the cations but also the activities of enzymes like alkaline phosphatase and creatinine kinase, which require these cations for optimal activity. To avoid contamination, blood collection tubes without anticoagulants or preservatives should be filled first, followed by heparinized tubes (if required), followed by EDTA tubes. If anticoagulants are used, it is important to ensure that the proper ratio of blood to anticoagulant is used. If very small blood samples are taken into tubes with anticoagulant, there may be a significant dilution of the blood sample, leading to erroneously reduced values for some analytes. Serum separator tubes are commonly used to separate serum from cells more easily in a blood sample. The separation is necessary to block the serum changes that would develop if cell metabolism were to continue. Separator tubes contain an impenetrable gel with a density intermediate between the cellular and serum components. When the sample is centrifuged, the gel forms a barrier between the cellular and serum elements, preventing metabolism effects. The samples with gel can be handled, centrifuged, and stored without removing the stopper, thereby reducing evaporation and the risk of aerosols. Most components of serum or plasma are unaffected by separator gels. A few therapeutic agents (tricyclic antidepressants and flecainide) have been found to adsorb to the gel, lowering their concentrations in serum, and if trace metal analysis is anticipated, it may be preferable to avoid gels, which could contain trace metal contaminants.

Tourniquets can make collection of blood easier at times, but the blood stasis they produce can lead to changes in the blood sample results. Tourniquet application results in water and electrolytes moving from the intravascular to the extracellular fluid space, causing an increase in the concentration of cells, proteins, and plasma components bound to proteins. Significant changes can begin in 3–4 minutes.

Variations from Hemolysis and Intravenous Fluids. Trauma to red blood cells during blood collection or transport can lead to hemolysis. The main cause of hemolysis is turbulent blood flow during sample collection, when blood moves either very slowly or too quickly through the needle. Blood drawn forcefully with a syringe or injected into collection tubes with too much pressure can lead to hemolysis as well. After the sample is drawn, excessive turbulence during transport can lead to hemolysis; this risk can be reduced by completely filling the specimen tubes.

Hemolysis is detrimental to serum chemistry analysis in two ways. First, the release of red cell contents falsely elevates the values of these components in serum; this is most evident with potassium and magnesium. Second, hemoglobin absorbs light over much of the light spectrum, so that hemolysis may interfere with many spectrophotometric measurements commonly used for other serum components.

Intravenous fluid contamination of blood samples can be a source of error for inpatients on intravenous therapy. Intravenous fluids commonly contain high concentrations of electrolytes, glucose, and drugs that can cause spurious increases in blood samples. Because contamination occurs when blood is drawn from a vein connected to the catheterized vein, it can be avoided by using a vein at some distance from the catheter site. Contamination of blood withdrawn near the catheter site can be reduced by discarding the first blood drawn equal in volume to that of the catheter.

Labeling Specimens. Proper labeling of the collected specimen may seem like the simplest of procedures, but it is one of the most common causes of laboratory error. It is important to label the specimen container with the correct name and identification number. In large animal hospitals, computer systems can provide preprinted labels with collection lists. A bar code can be placed on these labels with one or more of the following items: name, identification number, time specimen collected, tests required, name of clinician. Bar codes reduce clerical errors and can save considerable time if integrated to provide automated test requests.

Transportation, Centrifugation, and Storage. Local transport in a large hospital setting is usually rapid enough to avoid errors caused by delays in transport of whole blood prior to testing. One sample that will change appreciably with a delay of 1 hour is arterial blood for blood gas analysis. Such samples should be transported in an ice slurry and be tested as quickly as possible after collection. For glucose analysis, collecting with glycolytic inhibitors such as fluoride can prevent glucose metabolism in the sample. If serum separators or plain tubes are used, allow 30 minutes for clot formation to be complete before centrifugation. After centrifugation of plain tubes, serum should be separated quickly to prevent leakage of electrolytes, enzymes, and other small molecules from the cells.

Transportation to more distant sites like regional laboratories requires additional considerations to avoid errors. A few tests require whole blood, but for many tests serum or plasma should be separated from the cells, and the samples can be sent in insulated containers containing dry ice or ice packs.

Generally, centrifugation at 1,000–2,000 g for 5–10 minutes is sufficient to separate cells from serum. As indicated above, be certain that clotting is complete prior to centrifuging. With separator tubes, centrifuging with horizontal rotors is preferable to fixed angle–head rotors. With the latter, gaps can occasionally occur, allowing some contact between serum and cells.

Components of serum and plasma for many serum chemistry analyses are stable for 48–72 hours if stored at 4°C. For delayed testing of enzyme activities, hormones, and other small proteins, it is necessary to store the samples frozen. Care should be taken to avoid repeated thawing and freezing of specimens.

Rejection of Specimens. Each laboratory should establish a set of criteria for rejection of specimens so that erroneous results are not reported. Several problems warrant consideration for specimen rejection: inadequate or ambiguous specimen identification, specimen collected with inappropriate anticoagulant or preservative, inappropriate ratio of sample to preservative or anticoagulant, and significant hemolysis or turbidity of sample. If there is doubt about the validity of a laboratory result, the result should not be reported. Errors in laboratory results can lead to errors in treatment selection, which in turn can compromise the health of the patient.

Records of Reagent and Specimen Handling. The standard laboratory procedures section of the laboratory quality manual (see "Standard Analytic Procedures," below) should describe any particular conditions required for the reagents for a test, the specimen(s) required for each test, and any special considerations for specimen collection, transport, or stable storage.

Chain-of-Custody Considerations. In some situations where laboratory tests may have legal consequences (e.g., racetrack testing), specimen identification is required at every step of collection, transportation, and testing. A chain-of-custody form, like that in Figure 5.1, should be used for these samples. The process begins when a seal is placed on the specimen container at the time of sampling. Each person handling the specimen thereafter notes the date and time he or she receives the specimen and initials the form. This chain-of-custody process ensures that the laboratory results are from the correct specimen and therefore would be admissible in court if necessary.

LABORATORY SERVICES
Chain-of-Custody Form
(This form must remain with specimen until analysis is complete.)

Owner Name _____ Animal Name _____ Lab Number _____
Collection Date/Time _____ Collected by _____
Type of Specimen _____ Number of Specimens _____
Owner and/or Witness Signature(s) _____

TRANSPORTATION

Transported by Name/Date/Time	Received by Name/Date/Time	Seal Intact?
1.	1.	1.
2.	2.	2.
3.	3.	3.

TESTING

Specimen Opened by Name/Date/Time	Witnessed by Name/Date/Time	Seal Intact?

Figure 5.1. Example of a chain-of-custody form.

Laboratory Information Systems

One aspect of laboratory operations with important consequences for both quality and efficiency is the laboratory information system (LIS). The main function of the laboratory is to provide accurate information to its clients. The LIS must be structured and used with great care to ensure that information from the analysis of the specimens is integrated with the patient and owner information and transferred to the client quickly with minimal error. In addition to these operational requirements, the LIS can be designed to help with quality assurance and laboratory management functions.

Computer-assisted LISs have several quality assurance advantages over manual recording systems. Computerized systems reduce the number of manual transfers of patient demographic and test information, thereby reducing the time required for data management and the number of transcription errors. Computerized systems, by integrating patient identification, sample identification, tests requested, price lists, and test results, permit automation of many laboratory functions, including specimen tracking, laboratory section worklists, inventory control, and automated reporting and billing. Regardless of the type of data management system, the important first step in laboratory information management is to maintain a log that contains the date received, the identity of the patient, and the identity of the specimen and matches these to the tests requested and the specimen identification label. Some method of specimen tracking should be instituted to determine the stage of processing of any sample in the laboratory at any time. Laboratory worklists should be generated for each technologist or section to clearly identify the tests required on each set of samples. Reports should be printed so that the results are clear, with the appropriate reference ranges and abnormal values flagged for easy detection. Laboratory reports should be delivered in a timely manner; quick medical decisions and actions based on laboratory results are often crucial to the health of patients. Laboratory results can be delivered quickly by telephone, fax, or direct computer link. Abnormalities considered to be medically dangerous should be reported immediately by telephone or fax.

Continuous communication with clients is important to quality assurance. The laboratory should have personnel or readily available consultants who can quickly respond to questions on specimen collection or transport, turnaround time, costs, test characteristics, and test interpretation. A well-designed laboratory quality manual serves as an excellent resource for this purpose. Client feedback on accuracy, timeliness, and medical value of tests, as well as suggestions for new tests, should be actively sought in an effort to continuously improve the quality of service.

Computer-based LISs, due to their timesaving and error-reducing qualities, are becoming a more common means of handling information in veterinary laboratories. It is worthwhile to examine the features of a computer-based LIS to understand its potential role in quality assurance.

The LIS consists of hardware, operating system software, and applications (mainly database management) software. Each laboratory differs somewhat in its organization, size, complexity, mandate, and so on. The LIS should be structured to accommodate the unique organizational and operating needs of each laboratory.

MAIN FEATURES OF THE SYSTEM

The list of tasks that can be incorporated into the LIS includes patient identification, test order entry, specimen tracking, manual and instrument worklists, automated results entry through analyzer interfaces, manual results entry, results validation, quality control, report printing (local or remote), report faxing, electronic remote access to reports, integration of laboratory reports with hospital records, archiving of patient data, workload records generation, and billing.

PATIENT IDENTIFICATION

The patient and owner must be defined in the LIS before any tests can be run. This information can be entered into the LIS manually from a test request form, or it can be entered automatically, either electronically from another computer or from a card that has been prepared for hospital admitting.

The patient identification information (often referred to as patient demographics) usually consists of the following:

- Unique patient identification number

- Owner's name

- Sex of patient

- Date of birth of patient

- Species and breed of patient

- Referring veterinarian (or submitter of specimen) who will receive report

- Tentative diagnosis and/or brief history

TEST ORDER ENTRY

After the patient demographics have been entered, the order entry for tests requested must be entered and matched with the patient. Usually the information will be on a paper test request form that laboratory personnel must enter manually into the LIS. It is possible to program the system to do several checks on the data as they are entered in order to minimize errors. For example, the system can contain lists of valid tests for a given species, valid referring veterinarians, and valid test entry personnel; if the entered information does not match one of the entries in the valid lists, it is not accepted.

SPECIMEN IDENTIFICATION AND TRACKING

An identifying label must be placed on the specimen that contains patient identification information and the tests ordered. Most specimen labels have a specimen number as well, which allows the LIS to match the patient with the specimen and the tests requested. The specimen identification number can be printed on the label in Arabic numerals, as a bar code, or both. Bar codes are preferable because they decrease errors and save time, especially if bar coding is coordinated with automated instruments that read bar codes.

The specimen is often divided into aliquots for analysis in more than one laboratory or section of the lab. In this case, duplicate bar code labels can be printed, and the LIS can track each specimen or aliquot. In this way, laboratory personnel can check the system at any time to determine the location and stage of analysis of each specimen.

INTERFACES WITH ANALYTIC INSTRUMENTS

Increasingly, automated instruments are doing much of the testing in veterinary laboratories. Automation is desirable especially with high-volume tests. Interfacing the automated instruments to the LIS has several advantages. It eliminates most transposition errors and reduces time and labor costs associated with manual data recording, thereby improving test turnaround time. Interfacing involves a physical connection between the analytic instrument and the LIS, as well as interface software to allow data to flow between the instrument and the LIS. The interface allows the instrument to link the specimen and requested tests with the patient; many instruments accomplish this through the bar code on the specimen. Many interfaces allow for information transfer in one direction, from the instrument to the LIS. In this case the instrument reads the bar code and sends the test results to the appropriate patient file in the LIS. Some systems have bidirectional interfaces, allowing the instrument to read the specimen bar code and ask the LIS for tests requested on that particular patient's specimen.

The order in which the specimens are processed by an instrument is called the worklist. If there is no interface, the technologist must manually assign each specimen in the instrument to the specimen number in the LIS. Several approaches are used. The technologist can create a worklist manually on the LIS by entering the list of specimen numbers and matching them to specific instrument positions. In a second approach the specimen numbers are entered into the LIS, and the specimens are processed in precisely that order on the instrument. Another approach is that the computer automatically creates a worklist in order of specimen number or time of entry, and the technologist places the specimens into the instrument in the same order.

The instrument worklist is also useful for data validation. Results are examined before they are released, and if any are outside predetermined limits, the technologist can, for example, repeat the test, sometimes with dilution. Some instruments automatically dilute the specimen and retest it if it is outside the limits. The technologist then examines all results and selects those that are valid for release.

ENTERING RESULTS INTO THE SYSTEM

Results can be entered into the LIS either manually or automatically from an interfaced instrument. Manual entry is used in several situations: (1) if the test is not automated, (2) if the test volume is too small to justify interfacing, or (3) if abnormal results are repeated on different methods or instruments. Depending on the test volume, it is often valuable to generate a printed worklist manually so that results can be entered adjacent to specimen numbers.

When the results are manually entered into the LIS, it is advantageous to have a system that checks the data for abnormal limits, technologist validity, or other specified items in an effort to keep errors to a minimum. If considerable manual data entry is required, the software can be programmed to convert single keystrokes into commonly used words in the report. Despite these software checks and shortcuts, manual data entry is time-consuming and prone to error.

Automated data entry from interfaced instruments is preferable when it is feasible. It avoids transposition errors and is much faster. The results from the instrument are first validated by the technologist, and out-of-range results are checked, dilutions made, and samples rerun if necessary. Then the results are automatically downloaded into the LIS patient database, ready to report. The data checks outlined for manual entry apply to automated entry as well.

REPORTING RESULTS FROM THE SYSTEM

Laboratory results can be reported as paper reports that are mailed or telephoned to clients. Increasingly, results are being transported as electronic reports to other terminals or client computers or remote printers. In large institutions, like veterinary colleges, that have affiliated hospitals, electronic transmission of reports to remote terminals saves time and duplication of paper reports. The LIS can be programmed for automatic faxing of results to clients at predetermined intervals during the day, or the results can be transferred electronically from the LIS to the client's computer. Electronic transmission of reports and automatic faxing greatly reduce personnel time required for telephone reporting, and there are fewer transcription errors.

Paper reports are usually required for the permanent patient record, and if results are initially sent electronically, most laboratories send a follow-up paper report by mail to the referring veterinarian. The laboratory report usually contains the following information:

- Patient demographic information

- Veterinarian ordering tests

- Specimen collection date

- Time and date test was done

- Results of tests, with abnormal values flagged

- Reference ranges

- Interpretive, descriptive, or other comments, and diagnosis when appropriate

ARCHIVES AND DATA RETENTION

Although no general regulations apply to veterinary medicine, a useful guideline is to retain all test request forms and results for at least 5 years. The information may be useful for subsequent medical problems in a patient or for legal matters that may arise in relation to a case. The data can be stored in paper form or on microfiche, tape, floppy disks, or optical disks.

QUALITY ASSURANCE AND MANAGEMENT ASPECTS OF THE SYSTEM

Daily quality control information that supports the accuracy and precision of reported results can be automatically or manually entered into the LIS. The values of controls can be regularly evaluated for significant deviations beyond specified limits. This information may be required later for audit, regulatory, or legal issues. The LIS can report average turnaround times for specific tests to evaluate how well the laboratory is meeting its target values. The ordering frequency of the various tests provided by the laboratory can also be summarized by the LIS. This kind of information allows the laboratory management to evaluate the need for consumables, equipment, and personnel in the various sections of the laboratory more accurately and may identify inefficient sections or individuals. The test ordering patterns of specific clients may also be valuable for planning.

SECURITY OF LABORATORY INFORMATION

Computerized laboratory information systems must be designed with care to strike a balance between the somewhat conflicting goals of ready access to laboratory information and adequate security and data privacy. Several security features are common in an LIS. The LIS usually controls access with a user name followed by a password. The system can be programmed to change passwords regularly. User codes can be developed to limit LIS functions to various groups of users. Some people may be limited just to reading results, whereas others may be allowed to order tests and enter test results. Sensitive information related to, for example, potential legal cases may require a special access code to view.

For small laboratories, these types of security features are relatively easy to implement, but in larger institutional laboratories associated with animal hospitals or veterinary colleges, managing access to the LIS is a much more complex task and requires considerable care to maintain adequate security. New computer technology is increasing the need for care with security. Computer networks in large institutions and connections to the Internet provide potential international access to databases. This increased potential access will require continued care to avoid security breaks, malicious damage to data, and introduction of computer viruses into the system.

Standard Analytic Procedures

A continuously updated standard analytic procedures section of the laboratory quality manual is a central component of a good quality assurance program. Standardized procedures reduce variability, thereby supporting precision in measurements. The standard analytic procedures section should contain a thorough description of each procedure, with details about the specimen required, the equipment, the method, interfering substances, cross-reactions, medical use and reference values, special considerations about species or safety, records of analytic problems, and procedures used to solve the problems. An example of a typical page from the standard analytic procedures section is illustrated in Figure 5.2.

The adoption of Système International (SI) units for reporting results is another means to encourage consistency among laboratories (Appendix 2).

Standard Screening of Reports

Prior to reporting results from the laboratory, the reports should be checked very carefully for obvious errors and discrepancies. In a large, busy laboratory, errors occasionally are not detected with the standard internal control procedures, and sometimes errors occur at the report generation stage. The checking of reports can be done by a laboratory manager or a microbiologist, pathologist, or endocrinologist as he or she is interpreting the reports. The obvious errors that can be detected at this stage are results that are biologically impossible or extremely unlikely, based on past experience. For example, in a hematology laboratory, check that the hemoglobin is approximately one-third of the hematocrit, as expected; if not, is there a medical reason, or is there a problem with the red cell count? Is the plasma protein value slightly greater than the serum protein, as expected? In chemistry, are the urea and creatinine values consistent? Check extremely high values and 0 or undetectable values carefully. For example, is it biologically possible to get a serum potassium concentration of 19.8 mmol/L in a living dog, or could this be a urine sample that has been mistaken for a serum sample? In bacteriology, an *E. coli* sensitive to penicillin would be highly unlikely, warranting further investigation for a possible error in the procedure. And so on. Carefully checking results before they are released can detect a number of these types of errors.

Interpretation of Laboratory Tests

Results of laboratory tests, integrated with other clinical measurements, are used to make medical decisions. What is the diagnosis? Is a surgical or medical approach preferable for this problem? What is the prognosis? What therapy is most appropriate in this case? Should the therapy be altered for this patient? Answers to these and other medical questions often depend partly on laboratory results. For a medical decision to be optimally effective, the interpretation of test results must be valid. Valid test result interpretation requires confidence in the validity of the test

Procedure Name	Serum (Plasma) Glucose Concentrate
	Glucose Oxidase–Peroxide Method (GOD-PAP)
Procedure Principle	$\text{Glucose} + O_2 + H_2O \xrightarrow{glucose\,oxidase} \text{gluconate} + H_2O_2$
	$2H_2O_2 + 4 - \text{aminophenazone} + \text{phenol}$
	$\xrightarrow{peroxidase} 4\text{-}(p\text{-benzoquinone-monoimino})\text{-phenazone} + 4\,H_2O$
Specimen	Serum, EDTA plasma, or heparinized plama if separated from blood cells within 30 min of blood collection.
	Blood samples collected in sodium floride anticoagulant, which inhibits glycolysis, may be stored for a maximum of 24 hr prior to cell separation.
	Try to avoid excitement at blood collection—transient hyperglycemia. Glucose concentrations are stable for 7 days if sample stored closed at 4°C.
	Lipemia (common in diabetes mellitus) will lead to falsely increased values.
Reagents and Equipment	Reagent prepared from two solutions (Boehringer Mannheim):
	1. Buffer/enzymes/4-aminophenazone—dissolve 1 bottle in 100 mL distilled water (stable 5 weeks at 2–8°C).
	2. Phenol—as supplied (stable to expiration date at 2–8°C).
	Reagent prepared by pipetting 2.0 mL solution **2** into bottle **1** and mixing (stable 4 weeks at 2–8°C).
	Equipment—Hitachi 911.
Details of Procedure	See Hitachi 911 manual for instrument settings.
	Use calibrator for automated systems.
	Quality Control—pooled serum for precision, external standard for accuracy.
Interfering Substances	Uric acid at very high concentrations.
Reference Values	**Canine:** 3.3–5.6 mmol/L **Equine:** 3.6–5.6 mmol/L
	Feline: 3.3–5.5 mmol/L **Porcine:** 3.6–5.3 mmol/L
	Bovine: 1. 8–3.8 mmol/L **Ovine:** 1.2– 3.6 mmol/L
Medical Significance	**Persistent hyperglycemia**—diabetes mellitus, Cushing's, glucagonoma.
	Transient hyperglycemia—excitement, stress, hyperthyroid, and others.
	Hypoglycemia—β-cell tumor, hypothyroid, glycogen storage, ketosis (cattle), neonatal, drugs (insulin, o,p-DDD, salicylates).
Species or Breed Considerations	Transient hyperglycemia resulting from excitement or stress is common is dogs and cats and can be especially high in cats (i.e., 15–20 mmol/L).
References	Trinder P. *Ann Clin Biochem* 6:24, 1969.
	Hoffmeister H., Junge B. *Z klin Chem klin Biochem* 8:613, 1970.
Special Considerations	Solution 1 has azide as stabilizer; solution 2 is phenol—do not swallow either, and phenol is caustic on skin. If skin contact, flush with polyethylene glycol or copious water and consult physician.
Revisions and Problems Log	1996—no problems.
	May 24, 1997— "outside control limits." Fresh batch reagent—solved problem.

Figure 5.2. Example page of the standard analytical procedures section of the laboratory quality manual.

results and knowledge of the appropriate reference values, medical decision levels, and the analytic characteristics of the test.

Confidence in the validity or accuracy of test results depends on the quality assurance program of the laboratory doing the tests. Does the laboratory follow a set of quality assurance principles and procedures? Does the laboratory participate in an external quality assurance program to check the accuracy of its procedures? A rigorous quality assurance program is the best promoter of confidence in the validity of laboratory test results.

Interpretation of laboratory test results also requires knowledge of the analytic precision of the procedure used to generate the test result. A valid interpretation of laboratory tests requires knowing not only the reference values for the appropriate population and the medical decision levels selected for the variable but also the analytic precision of the test.

Determining the meaning of a laboratory test result is often a difficult task because of the many sources of uncertainty in the various steps involved in generating the result. The analytic characteristics of a test (e.g., precision and accuracy) deal with the uncertainties and errors that can occur in the analytic aspects of a test. The medical characteristics of a test (e.g., diagnostic sensitivity and predictive values, as discussed in Chapter 6) deal with the uncertainties and errors that can occur when a test result is applied to make a medical decision. In addition, the biological variation that occurs between animals and within the same animal over time contributes a preanalytic source of uncertainty (as in reference values).

In order to interpret laboratory test results rationally, these various sources of uncertainty and error must be considered together. The analytic precision and accuracy required for a specific test depend on the inherent biological variation of the variable in the population and on the specific medical decision to which the test results will be applied. An example will help illustrate the relationships.

If we wished to use serum thyroxin (T4) values in cats to make diagnostic decisions, the interpretation of a particular serum thyroxin value will depend on the **usual standard deviation** of the T4 assay at the critical **medical decision levels** for T4 in the cat. If you are considering hyperthyroidism as a possible diagnosis in a sick cat, and the laboratory reports reference values of 13–56 nmol/L for T4, how do you interpret a T4 result of 65 nmol/L? First, consider that most calculated reference ranges for healthy animals are based on expected values for the central 95% of the population. Two or 3 out of every 100 healthy cats (2.5%) are therefore likely to have T4 values above 56 nmol/L. Second, if you set the critical medical decision level of T4 for hyperthyroidism in cats at 57 nmol/L (i.e., a value equal to or exceeding 57 nmol/L is consistent with hyperthyroidism in a cat), then interpretation of a T4 of 65 nmol/L will depend on the precision of the T4 analysis. If the usual standard deviation of the T4 procedure indicates that 1 *sd* is 6.0 nmol/L at a mean of 65 nmol/L, then you know that 95% of the time a reported value of 65 nmol/L is somewhere in the range of 53–77 nmol/L (i.e., mean plus or minus 2 *sd*), and you know then that there is some likelihood that this cat's T4, although reported as 65, could be 53 and therefore normal. On the other hand, if the usual standard deviation of the T4 procedure at 65 nmol/L indicates that 1 *sd* is 3.5 nmol/L, then you know that 95% of the time a reported value of 65 is somewhere in the range of 58–73 nmol/L (i.e., mean plus or minus 2 *sd*), and you would have much more confidence that the reported value of 65 is abnormal (i.e., truly above 57) and consistent with the tentative diagnosis of hyperthyroidism. The main point here is that the same reported laboratory test value could have quite different medical interpretations, depending on the precision of the method.

As the example illustrates, the medical characteristics of a test and the analytic precision that your laboratory has for the test are interdependent, and both are essential to interpreting the result properly. The critical medical decision levels selected for a test can depend on the analytic precision of the analysis. If the T4 analysis in the above example was less precise (1 *sd* of 8 nmol/L), it may be preferable to change the critical medical decision level to 58 or 60 nmol/L if it is considered important to avoid too many false positive diagnoses.

A complete discussion of how test results are used to make medical decisions is beyond the scope of this book, but a few points are worth considering. Measures like diagnostic sensitivity, specificity, and positive predictive value, used to evaluate the medical value of a laboratory test (see Chapter 6), are valuable if you wish to use a test result as a screening test in a healthy population or if you wish to select a test to monitor a patient with a specific disease. These measures, however, are often of less value when you are faced with making a diagnosis in a specific patient. These measures are usually calculated for specific tests and/or diseases. The diagnostic situation with a patient requires that, based on the results of many clinical and laboratory results, you must determine to which of many possible diagnostic categories the patient belongs. Although Bayesian logic can be used for multiple tests and multiple diagnoses, the calculations often assume that the test results are independent of each other. This assumption is not valid for many groups of tests. If, on the other hand, the tests are treated as interdependent, then the calculations required for the Bayesian approach become extremely complex.

In most diagnostic situations, the various clinical and laboratory results must be integrated to find the appropriate specific diagnosis. The diagnostician could theoretically evaluate each test in turn by comparing each with its reference values. Diagnosticians, however, seem to integrate results in more of a parallel multidimensional fashion. If, for example, the critical medical decision levels of 5 out of 6 key tests for a diagnosis were reached, and the sixth value was only a couple of units away from the critical decision level, the diagnosis would likely be made. Rather than adhering strictly to every medical decision level, considering each test in turn, diagnosticians seem to use these levels as guides and to integrate the values of many tests together to arrive at a type of aggregate consensus view of which diagnosis is most likely, considering all of the clinical and laboratory information together. For very complex medical decisions requiring the consideration of large amounts of information, computer-assisted medical decision aids are being developed that also use methods that aggregate information in a parallel multidimensional fashion[14,15], similar to that used by experienced veterinary diagnosticians. Computer-assisted decision systems will likely be more routinely used for quality control and for the interpretation of test results in the future.

Chapter 6

___

Evaluating Laboratory Procedures

New or revised laboratory procedures are constantly being developed and are regularly introduced into the laboratory. New tests come to the attention of the laboratory either through in-house research activities or through professional journals, scientific or trade conventions, trade publications, or commercial reports. A preliminary judgment on the likely value of the new test can often be made from these sources. If the procedure looks promising, the laboratory should systematically evaluate it. New procedures supplied by commercial manufacturers should receive the same evaluation as those developed in the laboratory. A protocol similar to the following stepwise assessment is suggested to examine the practicality, the analytic characteristics, and the medical value of the new test procedure.

Evaluating the Practicality and Potential Value

Which species and which health problems does the test address? What will be the medical use of this procedure? Is it a diagnostic test, a prognostic test, a monitoring procedure, a screening test, or several of these? How is this new test likely to be better than existing tests? More accurate, more precise, more specific, more sensitive, or less costly? What are the specimen requirements, and do they pose a significant risk to the patient? Are the conditions required for specimen collection and transport realistic? What equipment is required? Is there sufficient personnel capability in the laboratory? What is the cost per test? Is the turnaround time reasonable? What are the reagent storage requirements? Does the test pose any safety risks? What workload can be expected? If only a few requests for a test are expected, would it be preferable to send them to a reference laboratory? (A laboratory cannot usually justify setting up a procedure that will be used only a few times per year. With low test volumes, the cost per test is usually high, and quality assurance is more difficult to maintain and more costly.)

If the answers to these questions are appropriate, do several dry runs or a feasibility study of the procedure. Assemble the materials and instruments and run through the new procedure once daily on 3 or 4 different days, using several random clinical specimens and controls in each run. These dry runs develop familiarity and permit a preliminary assessment of the procedure's practicality.

Evaluating the Analytic Characteristics

A method's performance is acceptable only if its analytic errors are small enough to permit valid medical decisions. Valid medical decisions require that the **total analytic error** for a procedure be less than the allowable error (as defined in Chapter 2). Method evaluation experiments are required to determine the analytic errors of the method and relate them to the medical requirements. Errors that affect the performance of a procedure may be either **random errors** or **systematic errors**.

Factors leading to random errors affect the precision of the measurement. Factors that can increase random errors include (1) temperature variations, (2) instrument instability, (3) variations in reagents and calibrators, (4) variations in technologists, and (5) variations in pipetting or timing. **Within-run variations** often result from variations in pipetting, temperature, or instrument stability. **Between-run variations** (on the same day) often result from recalibration differences, instrument variations, condition variations for controls, or staff fatigue. **Between-day variations** often result from changes in calibrators or reagents (new vials), instrument variations, or day-to-day staff changes.

Systematic error refers to error that is consistently in one direction or the other (i.e., consistently high or consistently low). A **constant systematic error** is one that is constant in size regardless of the concentration of the analyte. Constant systematic errors can be positive or negative and are independent of the concentration of the analyte. The following are common causes of constant systematic errors:

- An interfering substance in the reagents or in all of the samples, resulting in a false reading

- An interfering substance reacting with one or more of the reagents (lack of specificity)

- An interfering substance that blocks or reduces the reaction between the reagents and the analyte

- An interfering substance that breaks down the reagent, reducing its optimal concentration

- Improper blanking of the sample or reagents

A **proportional systematic error** is a systematic error that varies in size in proportion to the concentration of the analyte. The most common cause of a proportional systematic error is an incorrect amount of material in the calibrator.

All new procedures (or established procedures being adapted to a new instrument or applied to a new species) should be validated for the following **analytic characteristics:**

1. **Precision**—the random variation among replicate measurements

2. **Accuracy**—the systematic error between a measured value and the true value

3. **Detection limit** (sensitivity)—the least concentration of analyte detectable by the method

4. **Specificity**—the method's ability to measure only the analyte it was designed to measure

5. **Recovery**—the ability of a method to measure pure analyte added to sample material

6. **Reportable range**—the concentration range over which the method provides medically valid results

7. **Interference**—the effect of sample components on the accuracy of analyte measurement

In order for these characteristics and the error estimates to be valid, the operator must become familiar with the procedure, and the calibrators, controls, and reagents must be stable. For commercial materials, the manufacturer's expiration dates can usually be relied upon to ensure stability. For materials prepared in the laboratory, it is necessary to do a crossover study, comparing the results of patient samples with fresh and old calibrators to ensure their stability.

The various evaluation studies undertaken to determine analytic errors can be grouped as preliminary and final, as described in Table 6.1. The less expensive preliminary studies can be done first to avoid doing the more expensive final studies if the early ones indicate that the method has too great an error for valid medical use.

WITHIN-RUN PRECISION

Precision indicates the consistency with which a procedure will give the same value on repeated measurements of the same sample. Precision is the repeatability or reproducibility of a procedure and is measured by calculating the degree of variability around the central value of a procedure. **Within-run precision** measures the short-term variability among a set of repeated measurements of a sample on the same run of a procedure. A within-run precision study is simple, quick, and inexpensive and can therefore be the first means to assess the performance of a

Table 6.1. Evaluation studies for estimating different types of analytic errors

Type of Analytical Error Detected	Evaluation Study Required	
	Preliminary Assessment	Final Assessment
Random error	Within-run precision with pure materials and patient samples	Run-to-run precision with patient samples
Constant systematic error	Interference	Compare with standard method
Proportional systematic error	Recovery	Compare with standard method

Source: Adapted from Westgard et al.[10]

method. The within-run precision study should be done first with aqueous standards, if available, and repeated with controls in material similar to patient's samples. To determine within-run precision, analyze 15–20 replicates of 2 or 3 controls, each at different medical decision points (e.g., high, low, and normal). Calculate the mean, standard deviation, and coefficient of variation for each set of results. Compare the observed standard deviation (or coefficient of variation) with the standard deviation acceptable for the test relative to the medical needs. If the analytic error is greater than the allowable error, look for possible errors causing the imprecision. If these are not detectable, reject the procedure.

REPORTABLE RANGE, LINEARITY, AND SENSITIVITY

Prepare a set of samples containing known amounts of the analyte at increasing concentrations from zero to concentrations covering the range expected in clinical specimens. A set of aqueous standards and dilutions of analyte in sample material is usually used, as well as serum/reagent blanks. Analyze the samples and plot the observed values versus the known values. The analytic range and linearity can be assessed from the graph. Check that the limits of the linear range correspond to those claimed by the manufacturer. The reportable range is the concentration range over which the precision and accuracy are sufficient to provide medically valid results. The plot of observed values versus known concentrations, the **standard curve**, should ideally be linear, passing through the origin of the graph. A linear curve is usually necessary because the 2 or 3 standards or calibrators used when the method is run routinely assume a linear curve. If the relationship is not linear, the procedure will require several calibrators, especially in the areas of greatest curvature, for valid calibration throughout the range. The **analytic sensitivity**, or **detection limit**, indicates the least concentration of an analyte that can be detected by a procedure. The lowest concentration detected can be observed on the graph, but the sensitivity depends partly on the precision also. If the precision is poor at low concentrations, there will be little confidence in a given low value. (It is valuable to determine precision at low values that are important medically.)

ACCURACY AND RECOVERY

The **accuracy** of a procedure indicates its ability to measure the true value of an analyte. Because the actual true value cannot be known with absolute certainty, the true value is sometimes assumed to be the value determined on a standard reference method when using certified standards or calibrators. This type of comparative analysis—that is, the new method versus the standard reference method—can be done in the laboratory as a measure of accuracy. The methods are compared using regression analysis, *t*-tests, and correlation coefficients (see statistics textbooks for method details). External quality assurance programs (discussed in Chapter 4) are another measure of accuracy for a laboratory. External programs compare the value from your laboratory to the mean or median value of many other laboratories analyzing for the same analyte in aliquots of the same sample. In this comparison the mean value of the large number of laboratories is assumed to be the true value, or benchmark, by which your laboratory measures its accuracy.

Recovery, which measures the ability of the procedure to recover known amounts of an analyte, is also related to accuracy. To determine recovery, add known amounts of an analyte to clinical specimens and prepare a baseline sample with diluent or solvent in the specimen without the analyte. The volume of analyte added to the sample should be less than 10% of the total volume to avoid diluting the sample matrix. The baseline samples should be prepared with the same volume of diluent. The concentrations of analyte used should approximate the concentrations important for medical decisions. After analyzing the samples, subtract the baseline value from the other observed values to get the recovered values. Divide the recovered values by the amount originally added to each sample and multiply each by 100% to get the percent recovery. The average percent recovery from several samples, compared with the maximum possible (100%) recovery, provides a measure of accuracy. The percent recovery can be used to determine the proportional systematic error of the method. The percentage of proportional systematic error is the difference between the calculated percent recovery and 100% recovery. Proportional error can be compared with allowable error to assess its medical significance.

SPECIFICITY AND INTERFERENCE

The **specificity** of a procedure indicates its ability to measure only the analyte it is designed to measure. One common problem with specificity is cross-reactions with similar substances that would result in falsely elevated values for the analyte in question. Related to specificity is **interference**, which occurs when substances are present in specimens that bind to one or more reactants or, in a similar way, interfere with the reaction. Color and turbidity changes resulting from hemoglobin, bilirubin, or lipids in serum lead to similar problems in several chemical assays, resulting in falsely increased or decreased values (see Chapter 7, Table 7.1). All spectrophotometric methods should be checked for interference by hemoglobin, bilirubin, and lipids because of their common occurrence in blood samples. To assess interference, a study similar to a recovery study can be done, substituting the potential interfering substance (e.g., hemoglobin, bilirubin, lipid, anticoagulant, drug) for the analyte and expressing interference in terms of the observed values in the interference samples compared with the baseline samples. Constant systematic error can be determined from an interference study as the overall average difference between the baseline samples and the samples containing the interfering substance. This constant systematic error can be compared with the allowable error to judge the medical value of the method. Manufacturers of reagents for particular procedures often test for interfering substances; these should be noted and recorded in the standard analytic procedures section of the laboratory quality manual (see Fig. 5.2).

RUN-TO-RUN PRECISION

Run-to run precision, also called **between-run precision** or **day-to-day precision**, measures the day-to-day variability among repeated measurements of a sample on different days and different runs of a procedure. To determine run-to-run precision, on 15–20 different days analyze 2 or 3 controls, each at different medical decision points (e.g., high, low, and normal). The material must be known as stable for the 20-day period. Calculate the mean, standard deviation, and coefficient of variation for each set of results. Compare the observed standard deviation (or coefficient of variation) with the standard deviation that would be acceptable for the test relative to the medical needs. All method evaluation studies should evaluate precision at key medical decision levels. If the result is not acceptable, look for possible errors causing the imprecision. (If the procedure involves an instrument, check and verify the precision of the instrument before doing the run-to-run evaluation on the method.)

COMPARISON-OF-METHODS STUDY

The systematic error of a method can be determined by a comparison-of-methods study that uses patient samples. Results of patient samples analyzed on the test method are compared with results of the same samples analyzed by a standard or reference method. (Ideally, the standard or reference method should be known as accurate and precise, with little or no random or systematic analytic errors.) Differences between the results of the two methods are then considered as systematic errors of the test method. (The common practice of comparing a new method with the method in routine use in the laboratory must be interpreted cautiously if the routine method is not of reference quality).

A good comparison-of-methods study requires analyzing 50–100 patient samples. The samples should be carefully selected, with analyte concentrations distributed throughout the expected range, and should be from patients with various diseases. Hemolyzed, lipemic, or icteric samples should be included if they do not interfere in the comparison method. The samples should be analyzed in duplicate with each method. The test and comparison methods should ideally be run at the same time, but if this is not possible, samples should be stored to ensure their stability.

The systematic differences between the two methods are often assessed by calculating the **bias**, that is, by subtracting the mean result of the test method from the mean result of the comparison method.

$$\text{Bias} = \frac{\sum (y_i - x_i)}{n}$$ (Equation 6.1)

where y_i and x_i represent the analyte concentrations of the individual samples by the test method and the comparison method respectively.

The significance of the bias can be determined statistically using the *t*-test statistic. A *t* value can be calculated as follows:

$$t = \frac{\text{Bias} \times \sqrt{n}}{sd} \quad \text{where} \quad sd = \sqrt{\frac{\sum (y_i - x_i - \text{Bias})^2}{(n-1)}}$$ (Equation 6.2)

The standard deviation of the bias, represented as *sd,* indicates the random error between the two methods. To determine the statistical significance of the bias, calculate the *t* value as above, and compare it with the critical *t* value (from a statistics textbook) for the appropriate degrees of freedom. If the calculated *t* value exceeds the critical *t* value, a statistically significant bias exists between the two methods. However, to determine whether the systematic error is acceptable for the laboratory, a *t*-test is insufficient; for the systematic error to be judged acceptable, the **bias** must not exceed the allowable error (regardless of the statistical significance).

CORRELATION AND REGRESSION STATISTICS FOR METHOD COMPARISONS
The **correlation coefficient (*r*)** can be used to indicate that two methods correlate with one another, but it is not a measure of the agreement between the two methods. Two methods could give quite different results at a given concentration of analyte but have a high correlation if the results of both methods changed proportionately with increasing concentrations of analyte.

If two methods do correlate, the results of a method comparison study can be plotted as a straight line and expressed as a linear regression equation:

$$y_i = a + bx_i$$ (Equation 6.3)

where y_i is the value for the test method, x_i is the value for the comparison method, *a* is the *y* intercept, and *b* is the slope.

The slope, *b,* provides a measure of the proportionality between the methods. A slope of 1, indicating no proportional error, would be the optimal value. The *y*-intercept, *a,* provides a measure of constant error. The standard error of the regression (standard error of the estimate), $s_{y,x}$ indicates the random error between the methods. An estimate of the systematic error at any particular decision level can be obtained by substituting the decision level concentration for x_i in the regression equation above to give the test method's *y* value at this concentration. The systematic error at this level is the difference between the calculated *y* value and the decision-level *x* value.

For the error calculations above to be valid, several conditions are necessary. First, the range of concentrations must be wide. To check that the range is appropriate for error determinations from the regression equation, calculate the ratio of the standard deviation of the comparison method to the standard deviation of the test method. If the ratio is less than 0.2, the linear regression approach is suitable.[11] The regression equation must also be linear throughout the range of values. The data should be examined for outliers, and if they are present, the outlier samples should be retested with both methods to confirm that they are real. The cause of outliers should be investigated. Outliers can be removed statistically,[12] provided there is less than 1 per 40 sample comparisons. If there are more than 1 outlier per 40 samples and their cause cannot be determined and corrected, reject the procedure. If the above conditions cannot be met, there are other regression methods that may be more suitable.[11]

Evaluating the Medical Characteristics

MEDICAL JUSTIFICATION FOR A TEST

A decision to introduce a new test into a laboratory should include a consideration of the likely uses of the test. There are many medical reasons to develop and use a laboratory test. The following list includes the main uses. **Diagnosis** is perhaps the most important reason for testing; the test may help to detect, exclude, or confirm a disease. **Prognosis** can often be estimated from the results of one or more tests. **Monitoring** a patient with one or more tests is common and has several uses. The tests may allow determining the progression or regression of a disease, the changes in drug levels of a particular medication, or the response of the patient to a particular treatment. **Treatment decisions** may depend on test results. A surgical treatment, for example, may not be considered if the platelet count is low. **Screening** of healthy patients for a disease is another use for laboratory tests.

The medical reasons for introducing a new test are important considerations. The most desirable analytic, medical, and practical characteristics of a test vary somewhat, depending on the use of a test. Although the ideal test may be accurate, precise, inexpensive, safe, sensitive, and specific, with high predictive values, the ideal rarely occurs. The particular test characteristics that are of the most concern vary with the reason for the test. In the case of a screening test for a disease of low prevalence in a healthy population, attention will be focused on determining that the test is very sensitive, very specific, safe for the animal, and preferably inexpensive. In the case of a test used to monitor therapy with a very effective drug that has harmful side effects at high concentrations, attention will be focused on determining that the test is very precise and very accurate, to ensure that critical drug concentrations are not exceeded.

MEDICAL CHARACTERISTICS OF A TEST

To be medically valuable, the results of laboratory tests must provide the clinician or pathologist with information that is useful for medical decisions. A commonly used approach to assessing the medical value of a laboratory test is to determine its medical characteristics in relation to a disease: **diagnostic sensitivity, diagnostic specificity, positive predictive value, negative predictive value,** and **diagnostic accuracy (efficiency)**. These characteristics can be determined from data that describe the results of the test on two populations, one population known to be free of the disease and one population known to have the disease. The existence or nonexistence of the particular disease in the individuals of the two populations is based on an explicit set of criteria (a "gold standard"). The various medical characteristics of the test can then be calculated, as summarized in Table 6.2.

If you know that a patient has a specific disease, **diagnostic sensitivity** indicates the likelihood that the patient will be positive for the particular test. The **false negative rate** for a test is equal to 100% minus the sensitivity. For example, if 99% of dogs with diabetes mellitus have hyperglycemia, then hyperglycemia is a very sensitive test for diabetes mellitus. The false negative rate of 1% indicates that only 1 in 100 dogs with diabetes mellitus will not be hyperglycemic.

If you know that a patient is free of a specific disease, **diagnostic specificity** indicates the likelihood that the patient will be negative for a certain test. If hyperglycemia has a specificity of 90% for diabetes mellitus, then 90% of dogs without diabetes mellitus will not have hyperglycemia. The **false positive rate** for a test is 100% minus the specificity. In this example, the false positive rate would be 10% (100% – 90%), indicating that 10 in every 100 dogs without diabetes mellitus (healthy or with another disease) will be hyperglycemic.

Diagnostic accuracy (efficiency), because it provides a measure of all test results (positive or negative) that correctly classify patients as having or not having a disease, is considered a valuable measure by some investigators. The diagnostic accuracy of a test can be determined by the formula in Table 6.2 or by summing the sensitivity and specificity and then dividing by 2. If the sensitivity is 90% and the specificity is 86%, then the diagnostic accuracy is 88%, which would indicate a very good test. If the diagnostic accuracy is below 50%, the test is not likely to be very useful.

Table 6.2. Determining the medical characteristics of a test

	Number with the disease	Number without the disease	
Number with positive test	TP (True positives)	FP (False positives)	TP + FP
Number with negative test	FN (False negatives)	TN (True negatives)	FN + TN
Totals	TP + FN	FP + TN	

Diagnostic sensitivity is an estimate of the likelihood that a patient will be positive for the test when the disease is present.

Diagnostic sensitivity (expressed as a percentage) $= \dfrac{TP}{TP + FN} \times 100\%$

Diagnostic specificity is an estimate of the likelihood that a patient will be negative for the test when the disease is not present.

Diagnostic specificity (expressed as a percentage) $= \dfrac{TN}{FP + TN} \times 100\%$

Positive predictive value is an estimate of the likelihood that a patient with a positive test has the disease.

Positive predictive value (expressed as a percentage) $= \dfrac{TP}{TP + FP} \times 100\%$

Negative predictive value is an estimate of the likelihood that a patient with a negative test does not have the disease.

Negative predictive value (expressed as a percentage) $= \dfrac{TN}{TN + FN} \times 100\%$

Prevalence is an estimate of the frequency of the disease in a population at a point in time.

Prevalence (expressed as a percentage) $= \dfrac{TP + FN}{TP + FP + TN + FN} \times 100\%$

Diagnostic accuracy (efficiency) is an estimate of the likelihood that a patient is classified correctly as diseased or not diseased.

Diagnostic accuracy (efficiency) expressed as a percentage $= \dfrac{TP + TN}{TP + FP + TN + FN} \times 100\%$

Both sensitivity and specificity help evaluate a test and give some indication of the expected false negative and false positive rates for the test, but they evaluate the test in patients already known to have or not have a specific disease. In medicine, however, we are usually more interested in what a test result means in a patient not known to have a particular disease.

The **positive predictive value** of a test is a more useful measure because it provides an estimate of the percentage of patients who are likely to have a specific disease if they are positive for the test. If hyperglycemia has a positive predictive value of 50% for diabetes mellitus, this indicates that 50% of dogs with hyperglycemia have diabetes mellitus. One important consideration with regard to positive predictive value is its dependence on the prevalence of the disease in the population of concern. The higher the prevalence of the disease, the better the positive predictive value. When the positive predictive value is determined on a sample of animals selected because of signs suggesting that they may have a certain disease, the predictive value may be quite high (the sample may contain animals with diseases other than the one being studied but with relatively few healthy animals); however, when the test is applied to the population at large, in which there is a much larger proportion of healthy animals, the prevalence of the disease will be much lower, and the predictive value may be very low and of limited use.

In order to calculate sensitivity, specificity, and predictive values, a test result must be scored as positive or negative. Many tests are measured on continuous scales, and the location of the lines drawn on these scales to separate positive from negative for a test have considerable influence on the sensitivity, specificity, and predictive values. For example, if we had an ideal diagnostic test for acute pancreatitis in the dog, test results on a population of dogs would look similar to those in Figure 6.1. The ideal test clearly separates animals with the disease from animals without it. The sensitivity is 100%, and the specificity is 100%. There is no overlap of values and no false positives or false negatives. In this ideal situation, the **medical decision level** could be set at 810 units/L for this test; the line labeled *a* in Figure 6.1, drawn on the measurement scale at 810 units, clearly separates the groups.

Unfortunately, the ideal test is rare in medicine. For most diagnostic tests, there is usually some overlap between animals with the disease and animals without, as illustrated in Figure 6.2. Determining the medical decision level or cutoff value in this situation is more problematic. A cutoff point at 810 units/L (labeled *a* in Figure 6.2) makes the false negative and false positive rates approximately equal. If the cutoff point is moved to point *b* in the figure, nearly all dogs with pancreatitis will have a positive test, but many dogs without pancreatitis will also have a positive test. In other words, moving the cutoff point to *b* greatly increases the sensitivity of the test, but at the expense of the specificity. If the cutoff point is moved in the opposite direction, to *c,* then almost every dog without pancreatitis will have a negative test (a very specific test), but many dogs with pancreatitis will be missed (loss of sensitivity).

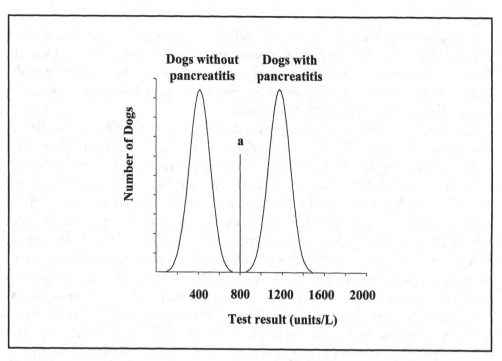

Figure 6.1. An ideal diagnostic test for acute pancreatitis would have values distributed in two distinct groups with no overlap between the groups and no false positive or false negative results.

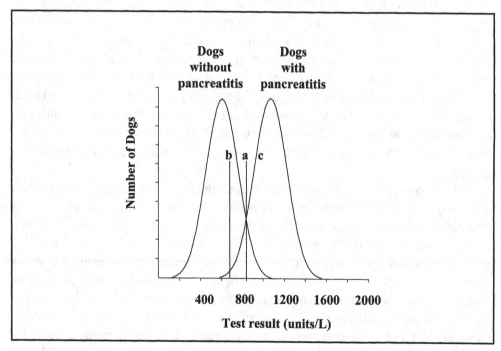

Figure 6.2. The usual diagnostic test for acute pancreatitis has values distributed in overlapping groups with false positive and false negative results dependent on the location of the cutoff point.

Selecting the location of the cutoff point results in trade-offs. The main considerations are the consequences of false negative or false positive results. If it is serious to miss the diagnosis and not treat the disease (especially if the treatment will not harm dogs without the disease), then move the cutoff point toward greater sensitivity (to the left in Figure 6.2). If it is not too serious to miss the diagnosis and leave the disease untreated (especially if the treatment also has some undesirable side effects), it may be preferable to move the cutoff point toward greater specificity (to the right in Figure 6.2). This would lead to making the diagnosis only in those animals with a high likelihood of having the disease.

Serum lipase activity in dogs is an example of this situation. Increased serum lipase activity is used as a diagnostic test for acute pancreatitis in dogs. Although dogs with acute pancreatitis usually have elevations in serum lipase activity, mild elevations in serum lipase can occur with other factors, including renal disease or prerenal problems, resulting in a reduced glomerular filtration rate; some hepatic diseases; or corticosteroid therapy. Serum lipase activities in dogs can be grouped into three categories, with distributions approximately similar to those depicted in Figure 6.3. A cutoff value of 1,200 units/L would provide a very specific test with few false positives, but it would be insensitive—the cases of pancreatitis with values between 600 and 1,200 would be missed. Because the consequences of leaving pancreatitis untreated can be serious, if the lipase value is between 600 and 1,200 units/L, additional or repeated tests will often be necessary to decide which of several possible diagnoses is most appropriate. Most medical diagnostic problems require considering more than a single test result.

Calculating the sensitivity, specificity, predictive values, and diagnostic accuracy of a test provides a set of measures on which to judge the medical value of a test. These characteristics help decide whether or not the test should be used routinely in a laboratory, especially when the individual test is likely to be used for monitoring, screening, or treatment decisions. It is important, however, to emphasize that these measures are often of limited value when you are faced with making a diagnosis in a sick animal. The sensitivity, specificity, and predictive values are

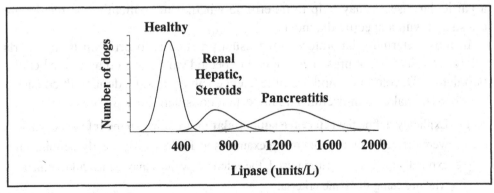

Figure 6.3. Approximate distributions of serum lipase activities in three populations of dogs.

usually determined for a specific test (or two) and a specific disease (or two). In many diagnostic situations, however, you are faced with the results of many tests and must decide to which of several possible diagnostic categories the patient belongs (as in the example above, with a lipase value between 600 and 1,200). The predictive value approach can be applied to situations with multiple tests and multiple diseases, but often either the assumptions required for these types of applications are not tenable or the calculations required become too complex to be practically feasible. The section "Interpretation of Laboratory Tests" in Chapter 5 addresses these issues further.

Setting goals for the medical characteristics of a test is difficult to generalize because the goals for particular tests depend somewhat on the intended medical use of the test (e.g., diagnosis, prognosis, screening). Also, the prevalence of certain diseases varies considerably with the geographic location, the type of practice clientele, and other factors. The medical characteristics of a test that are adequate in a region of high disease prevalence may not be adequate in a region of low disease prevalence. Determining the medical characteristics of laboratory tests in each context is therefore important. These values serve as important baseline measures to evaluate improvements in the sensitivities, specificities, and predictive values of new or revised tests.

REFERENCE VALUES

The usual first step in interpreting laboratory results is a comparison of the patient's results to a set of **reference values**, that is, the range of expected values for a defined subpopulation. We sometimes restrict the definition of "reference values" to the expected values in a comparable healthy population. Comparing the condition of the animal patient with what is expected in the healthy population helps us to decide whether the animal is healthy and, if not, whether the changes observed help lead us to one or more possible diagnoses.

Reference values developed for subpopulations other than healthy ones can also be helpful for comparisons with a patient's test results. The reference population could be healthy, diseased, or both, depending on the goal of the medical decision. Comparisons of a patient's values with values previously observed in animals with a particular disease may help to determine whether the patient's test results are consistent with a specific diagnosis.

In most veterinary laboratories, the usual practice is to print on their reports reference values that represent a range of expected values in a comparable healthy population. Development and use of reference values must be done with considerable care to make them useful. The important considerations are these:

1. Explicitly define the **reference subpopulation** from which the reference values were derived, as illustrated in the examples in Table 6.3. By clearly defining and explicitly stating the criteria used, the reference values may be useful to others who are using the same criteria.

Table 6.3. Examples of explicit definitions of reference subpopulations.

Factor	Reference Subpopulation A	Reference Subpopulation B	Reference Subpopulation C
Species	Canine	Canine	Bovine
Breed	All breeds	All breeds	Holstein
Age	>0.5 years	<0.5 years	>2 years
Sex	Female and male	Female and male	Female
Health status	Healthy[a]	Healthy[a]	Healthy[a]
Other	NA	NA	Postpartum <30 days

[a]"Healthy" indicates that neither the owner nor the veterinarian found behavioral or physical abnormalities that suggested illness, and the temperature, heart rate, and respiratory rate were within existing reference intervals.

2. The specimens, analytic methods, and quality control procedures used to derive the reference values should be explicit, so that others know the conditions under which the reference values are valid.

3. Develop the reference values with as large a sample as possible. Minimum numbers recommended vary from 40 to 100. The key point is that the larger the sample, the more likely it is that the reference values represent the population.

4. Examine the data from the reference population and discard any outliers that are clearly due to errors.

5. Calculate the limits of the reference values. The limits of values used as the reference values for a population have varied from the entire range observed, the mean $\pm$ 2 *sd,* or an interpercentile interval. An interval that is commonly used is the central 95% interval bounded by the 2.5 and 97.5 percentiles. One advantage to using an interpercentile interval like the central 95% interval is that it does not require the assumption of a Gaussian distribution.

6. The sick animal that is being tested should fit the criteria of the reference subpopulation. If, for example, the values from a sick 3-month-old dog were compared with reference values from subpopulation A in Table 6.3, errors could be made in the interpretation of the hematocrit, the serum protein concentration, and other variables that tend to differ between young dogs and adults.

Reference values commonly used in veterinary laboratories are often restricted only to species. They are assumed to represent all breeds, ages, and sexes within the particular species. This assumption is valid only if the reference values were derived from a population in which there was ample representation of all ages, breeds, sexes, and so on. Often this broad representation is difficult to achieve practically when reference populations are selected. Therefore, assumptions about representation are required with the use of most broad species-based reference ranges.

There are sometimes advantages to having reference values subcategorized according to age, sex, breed, or other characteristics (e.g., groups B and C in Table 6.3). Reference values representing a more limited subpopulation will show less biological variation and have a narrower range, thereby being more sensitive for detecting changes in sick animals. Although subcategorizing reference values for many of the conceivable specific groups such as age, sex, breed, or others would be impractical and expensive, subcategorized reference values would be beneficial for certain subpopulations in which several variables are likely to differ significantly from the larger population.

Reference values partitioned for age would likely be beneficial for neonatal and/or young animals in most species. Several of the variables regularly measured to assess health differ considerably in young versus adult animals. For example, young animals tend to have smaller red blood cells (RBCs), lower hematocrit values, lower RBC mean corpuscular volumes, and slightly lower serum iron concentrations, all of which could have a significant effect on an evaluation of possible diseases characterized by an anemia. Plasma and serum protein concentrations, serum phosphorus concentrations, and the activities of alkaline phosphatase, sorbitol dehydrogenase, and gamma glutamic transaminase in serum differ significantly between young animals and adults of certain species.

Specialty practices may find it useful to have reference values defined for more-specific subpopulations that are commonly addressed in their practice. For example, reference values similar to those of group C in Table 6.3 may be useful in a large-animal practice that deals exclusively with dairy herds.

Computerized laboratory information systems can be programmed to select and print the appropriate reference values for age, breed, or other properties on the report, depending on the patient identification data logged with the sample. The electronic system can also be programmed to flag results that differ from the reference ranges with, for example, an "H" for "high" and an "L" for "low," which is convenient for those interpreting the report.

We routinely work with reference ranges for individual variables of a population, yet the common clinical situation is to consider several test results together for interpretation and a decision. The possibility of comparing a multidimensional set of patient values with a corresponding multidimensional reference range is appealing.[13] The complex nature of developing multivariate reference ranges requires the use of a computer. The relative ease of integrating data for medical decisions by using fuzzy logic systems[14] suggests that they may be useful tools for developing multidimensional reference ranges.

Documenting the Procedure and Informing Clients

After the analytic and medical characteristics of a new test have been determined and found to be acceptable, the procedure should be documented in the laboratory quality manual, internal quality control limits should be established, and the staff should be trained on the procedure.

All clients should be informed about the availability and features of the test. Each laboratory should have a pamphlet or booklet for clients that lists each test, the specimen requirements, expected turnaround time, cost, reference values, the scheduling of tests (which are available for emergency purposes and which are available daily, weekly, or otherwise), and the location of testing (in-house testing or testing by a referral laboratory).

Chapter 7

Laboratory Choices and Point-of-Care Testing

Deciding which tests to run in a practice laboratory and which to send to a full-service diagnostic laboratory depends on many factors, several of which relate to quality assurance. Every veterinary practice should have some capability for laboratory testing with a good microscope, a microhematocrit centrifuge, a standard centrifuge, a refractometer, and the stains and supplies necessary to do a urinalysis, parasite testing, examination of a blood smear, dry strip analysis for serum urea and blood glucose, and cytological examination of body fluids and tissue aspirates. This range of tests, and in some practices a greater range, may be routinely run in-house. In other practices they may be run only for emergency or out-of-hours situations if a referral laboratory is nearby. The size of a practice and the resultant test volume dictate which tests should be run routinely in-house and which should be sent to a referral laboratory. The proximity of the referral laboratory and the availability of rapid courier services are also important considerations.

Chemistry

Small serum chemistry test units are available for blood chemistry analyses in a practice setting. These instruments require personnel with training and experience in both chemistry methods and quality control procedures and can be cost-effective in a large practice with large test volumes. Valid results with these instruments cannot be assured unless they are regularly calibrated and controlled, as outlined in Chapter 4. If the test volumes are low, the aggregate cost of labor, depreciation, and quality assurance procedures can often render the cost per test too high to be feasible. Compromising on the quality assurance procedures to save on costs is likely to increase errors and thereby erode confidence in the accuracy and value of the results. Unless test volumes are high and quality assurance procedures are regularly followed in a practice laboratory, most chemistry analyses should be sent to a large diagnostic laboratory, which can usually provide a greater variety of tests, better test precision and accuracy, and a lower cost per test.

An optimal condition for chemical analyses includes serum or plasma separated from cells quickly after blood collection and free of interfering substances. Hemolysis, icterus, lipemia, certain drugs, and anticoagulants are the most common substances that can interfere with chemical procedures, causing errors in test results. The type of error caused by the interfering substance (false increase or false decrease) depends on the method used for the particular assay and may therefore vary from one laboratory to another. It is helpful for each laboratory to summarize in chart form, as a quick reference for personnel, the main interference problems with procedures, as illustrated in Table 7.1. Potentially spurious results due to interference should be clearly flagged on the report form. Lipemia is commonly troublesome in dogs. In vivo methods, like fasting for 24 hours or 100 IU/kg of sodium heparin IV 15 minutes prior to sampling, often eliminate the problem. Separating the lipid fraction from serum by cooling and/or centrifugation may clear the sample, but the concentrations of analytes of interest may be altered by partial binding to the separated lipids.

Hematology

Routine hematological testing in a practice laboratory could include determining the packed cell volume (PCV) for red cells, the total plasma protein concentration on a refractometer, and examination of a blood smear. The blood smear, provided it is made properly with a large monolayer region, can be used to make an estimate of the number of total white blood cells (WBC); the number of platelets; the morphologic changes in red cells, white cells, and platelets; and occasionally the presence of microorganisms. Quantitative blood cell counts can be obtained with a hemocytometer, but the procedure is time-consuming, and the results are not very precise. Automated blood cell counting and related analyses available in a referral hematology laboratory can provide more information that will be more accurate, more precise, and more rapid.

Evaluation of a blood smear for cell morphologic changes, differential cell counts, and parasites is often critically important to medical decisions and must therefore be as accurate as possible. Blood cell characteristics vary considerably among the various animal species, so morphological assessments from automated counters calibrated for one species are of limited value for other species. Microscopic evaluations of blood smears are therefore essential in a veterinary hematology laboratory. To be accurate, a microscopic blood smear evaluation must be done by an experienced individual who has been well trained with examples from all of the

Table 7.1. Effects of hemolysis, icterus, or lipemia on serum chemical analyses

	Hemolysis		Icterus		Lipemia	
	False Increase	False Decrease	False Increase	False Decrease	False Increase	False Decrease
Total bilirubin	✓				✓	
Bile acids		✓			✓	
Total protein	✓		✓			✓
Albumin	✓					✓
Sodium						✓
Calcium					✓	
Phosphorus	✓				✓	
Glucose					✓	
Creatinine				✓		
Cholesterol				✓		
Creatinine phosphokinase	✓					
Alkaline phosphatase		✓				
Gamma glutamic transferase		✓				✓
Alanine aminotransferase	✓					✓
Aspartate aminotransferase			✓			✓
Amylase		✓			✓	
Lipase		✓			✓	

animal species that they will be expected to evaluate. If your facility does not have individuals trained on the species concerned, the smears can be examined and scored, with duplicates forwarded to a referral laboratory for an accurate comparative evaluation. By repeating this comparative evaluation and providing appropriate training, the practice laboratory can develop the expertise to evaluate blood smears of new species. Blood smears should be evaluated systematically with a checklist to ensure that all significant changes are noted. Smears should be evaluated at low magnification for changes in cell distribution (e.g., agglutination) and at oil-immersion magnification for differential counts and cell morphology. Differential white cell counts should be reported as absolute counts rather than as percentages, to avoid misinterpretation of relative changes in white cells. Total WBC counts with automated cell counters are usually 2–3 times more precise than manual counts using a hemocytometer. Falsely increased total WBC counts are often the result of aggregated platelets, large platelets, or inadequate lysing of RBCs. Falsely decreased total WBC counts can result from white cell clumping. Checking the blood smear carefully can often prevent reporting these types of errors in WBC counts. Automated blood cell counters must be calibrated for each of the various animal species to avoid errors due to the considerable variation in cell size among several species.

Hematology laboratory personnel should be trained to recognize the presence of a leukemia or abnormal leukocytes, erythrocytes, or platelets on a blood smear. Malignant neoplasms, for which subclassification may be valuable for prognostic or therapeutic decisions, should be sent to a referral laboratory for classification by a veterinary pathologist.

Accurate evaluation of bone marrow samples also requires considerable experience. If your laboratory has little experience with marrow evaluations, it is usually preferable to send samples to a referral laboratory to be evaluated by a trained clinical pathologist.

Coagulation

Accurate assessment of coagulation problems usually requires sending samples to referral laboratories that are equipped and experienced with these specialized assays. Sample management is extremely important to the accuracy of many coagulation tests. It is preferable to contact the referral laboratory for details on sampling, storage, or transportation of specimens required for coagulation tests.

Cytopathology and Parasitology

Cytopathologic evaluations of fluid and tissue aspirates, and examination of feces and other sites for parasites, can provide valuable diagnostic information. Valid interpretations of these samples require adherence to standard procedures, internal controls, and periodic audits as outlined in Chapter 4. To become proficient in cytopathologic evaluation and accurate parasite identification requires considerable training and experience. The practice of sending duplicate samples to a referral laboratory for a period of time can help laboratory personnel develop this proficiency. If a referral laboratory is nearby, it may be more cost-effective to routinely send these samples there for analysis. Referral laboratories often have well-trained and experienced pathologists and parasitologists on their staff who are proficient with these procedures. Periodic evaluation of cytopathologic and parasitologic tests by an external quality assurance program is a valuable check on the accuracy of the laboratory's procedures.

Bacteriology, Histopathology, and Therapeutic Drug Analysis

Most procedures involving bacteriology, histopathology, and therapeutic drug analysis require specialized and expensive equipment and should be sent to a referral laboratory with experience and expertise in these disciplines. They are likely to have good quality assurance procedures that ensure accurate and precise results.

Point-of Care Testing

The ability to do laboratory testing during a patient's visit to a clinic (rapid turnaround time) is a major motivation for point-of-care (POC) testing. Time delays and sample handling are minimized. These apparent benefits, however, create potential problems with the quality of results. The context and focus of attention with POC testing differs significantly from that in the laboratory. Personnel doing POC testing want results that can be used quickly for patient care, and there may be inadequate attention to analytical procedures, quality control, and data recording, which are routinely used in the laboratory. The laboratory qualifications of the individual doing the test may be inadequate to recognize problems with the test. Performance of quality control measures may be absent or inadequate; in some cases the test result may be acted on before any quality control checks have verified the validity of the result.

Sometimes POC instruments have built-in "electronic quality control," and some people have suggested that little additional quality control is necessary with these systems. However, instrument malfunction is one of the main reasons for quality control. If an instrument has electronic quality control, how well is the quality control system working if the instrument is malfunctioning? There is no doubt that electronic quality control is helpful for monitoring the performance of the instrument readout device, but electronic quality control cannot deal with the quality of all of the other steps in the preanalytic, analytic, and postanalytic aspects of laboratory testing. Good internal and external quality assurance programs and standard laboratory procedures, as described in Chapters 4 and 5, are necessary to ensure the quality of laboratory results.

If POC testing is used, some method must be implemented to ensure that the data are properly recorded and flow to the same places (clinician, hospital record, and so on) as if they had originated in the laboratory. This is especially important in large institutional laboratories associated with an animal hospital.

Tests of low complexity, as defined by the CLIA regulations, are suitable for POC testing. These include urine chemistry (dipstick or tablet-based urine chemistry), urine specific gravity (refractometer), fecal occult blood, hematocrit (centrifuge), hemoglobin, and blood glucose. Additional tests that may be considered are blood gases and electrolytes (sodium, potassium, and calcium), using the newer small portable analyzers for these tests. However, the potential quality control, supervision, and data integration problems discussed above should be addressed before adopting these latter POC procedures.

Veterinary Quality Assurance Programs

Veterinary Laboratory Association Quality Assurance Program®

The Veterinary Laboratory Association Quality Assurance Program® (VLAQAP) is an external quality assurance (proficiency testing) program provided by Diagnostic Chemicals Limited (DCL) in conjunction with the Atlantic Veterinary College (AVC). Modules are available each quarter and include chemistry, hematology, endocrinology, therapeutic drug monitoring, serology/immunology, bacteriology, parasitology, and histopathology. Each laboratory can select the combination of modules that meets its needs. All results are confidential. Each participating laboratory receives quarterly graphical reports, showing its individual results in relation to the participating group results, which are categorized by method and instrument when appropriate. There is a detailed descriptive review by an academic specialist for the results of hematology, parasitology, histopathology, and bacteriology. For additional information, contact

Diagnostic Chemicals Limited
West Royalty Industrial Park
Charlottetown, PEI Canada CIE 1BO
Telephone: (800)-565-0265 or (902)-566-1396
Fax: (902)-566-2498
Web site: www.dclchem.com
E-mail: vqap@dclchem.com

National Veterinary Services Laboratory

The National Veterinary Services Laboratory (NVSL) offers training for certification for running, interpreting, and reporting results of tests for equine infectious anemia (EIA), avian leukosis, and bluetongue virus. These programs require state approval or designation as a laboratory to run the tests. For additional information regarding NVSL training programs and certification for EIA, avian leukosis, and bluetongue virus testing in the United States, contact

> National Veterinary Services Laboratory
> P.O. Box 844
> Ames, IA 50010
> USA
> Telephone: (515)-239-8501

For information regarding EIA and bluetongue virus testing in Canada, contact

> Centre for Animal and Plant Health
> 93 Mount Edward Road
> Charlottetown, PEI
> Canada CIA 5TI
> Telephone: (902)-368-0950

American Association of Veterinary Laboratory Diagnosticians, Inc.

The American Association of Veterinary Laboratory Diagnosticians, Inc. (AAVLD), has an accreditation program for government and educational institutional diagnostic laboratories but does not yet accredit private or commercial laboratories. Its program covers self-evaluation, assessment of facility, equipment, personnel, quality control and quality assurance, operations, reporting, and recommendations for improvement. Minimum standards have been developed for anatomic pathology, toxicology, and serology. For additional information, contact

> American Association of Veterinary Laboratory Diagnosticians, Inc.
> CVDLS, SVM, UC Davis
> P.O. Box 1522
> Turlock, CA 95381
> USA

Endocrine Quality Assurance Program

Endocrine Quality Assurance Program (EQUAS) is a proficiency testing program directed by Dr. R. F. Nachreiner and sponsored by Daniels Pharmaceuticals and Diagnostic Products Corporation. Several endocrine tests are available for several species, and proficiency testing samples are sent each quarter. Participating laboratories receive reports showing individual results (categorized by method and/or instrument) in relation to peer group results. For additional information, contact

Endocrine Diagnostic Section
Animal Health Diagnostic Laboratory
P.O. Box 30076
Lansing, MI 48909-7476
USA
Telephone: (517)-353-0621

Appendix 2

Conversion of Units

Conversion of Conventional Units to Système International (SI) Units

Analyte	Conventional Unit ×	Conversion Factor	SI Unit
Blood cells	cells/μL	10^6	cells/L
Enzymes	IU/L	0.017	μkat/L[a]
Amylase	Somogyi units/dL	1.85	IU/L
Lipase	Cherry-Crandall units/mL	278	IU/L
Albumin	g/dL	10	g/L
Ammonia	μg/dL	0.554	μmol/L
Base excess	mEq/L	1	mmol/L
Bicarbonate	mEq/L	1	mmol/L
Bile acids	μg/mL	2.45	μmol/L
Bilirubin	mg/dl	17.1	mmol/L
Calcium	mg/dL	0.01	mmol/L
Carbon dioxide (total)	mEq/L	1	mmol/L
Chloride	mEq/L	1	mmol/L
Cholesterol	mg/dL	0.026	mmol/L
Cortisol	μg/dL	27.6	mmol/L
Creatinine	mg/dL	88.4	μmol/L
Fibrinogen	mg/dL	0.01	g/L
Folate	ng/mL	2.27	nmol/L
Globulins	g/dL	10	g/L
Glucose	mg/mL	0.055	mmol/L
Insulin	μIU/mL	0.0417	μg/L
Iron	μg/L	0.179	μmol/L
Magnesium	mg/dL	0.41	mmol/L

(continued)

Conversion of Conventional Units to Système International (SI) Units *(continued)*

Analyte	Conventional Unit ×	Conversion Factor	SI Unit
PCO_2	mm Hg	0.133	kPa[b]
PO_2	mm Hg	0.133	kPa[b]
Phosphate	mg/dL	0.323	mmol/L
Potassium	mEq/L	1	mmol/L
Protein	g/dL	10	g/L
Sodium	mEq/L	1	mmol/L
Urea	mg/dL	0.357	mmol/L

[a]1 katal (1 mol/sec) is the suggested unit for reporting enzyme activity, but most laboratories report activity as IU/L (1 μmol/min).
[b]kPa, kilopascal.

Glossary

accuracy–the systematic error between a measured value and the true value.

allowable error–the maximum error allowed in an analytic procedure for its test results to be medically useful.

analytic error–see *total analytic error*.

CLIA–Clinical Laboratory Improvement Amendments of 1988; a set of federal regulations governing the operation of human health laboratories in the United States.

coefficient of variation (CV)–a measure of variation relative to the mean, in which the standard deviation is divided by the mean and multiplied by 100%.

confidence interval–a range of values around a statistic, which has a known probability of containing the true population value.

constant systematic error–a systematic error that is constant in size and independent of the concentration of the analyte.

control limits–limits within which control values for the laboratory procedure must be for the patient sample results to be considered valid.

degrees of freedom–the number of independent observations in a set of observations.

detection limit–the least concentration of an analyte that can be detected by a procedure.

diagnostic sensitivity of a test–the likelihood that a patient known to have a disease will be positive for its test.

diagnostic specificity of a test–the likelihood that a patient known not to have the disease will be negative for its test.

external quality assurance (proficiency testing)–a monitoring system using unknown samples provided by an external agency that analyses the results of all participants to evaluate the accuracy of each participant's laboratory procedures.

interference–the effect of sample components on the accuracy of analyte measurement.

internal quality audit–a periodic random sampling of previous cases evaluated for quality.

internal quality control–a monitoring system using control materials to verify the acceptability of patient sample results.

laboratory quality manual–a manual describing the goals, policies, and procedures necessary to implement a quality assurance program, as well as the results of internal and external monitoring activities that document the quality of results.

mean–the sum of all the values of a data set divided by the number of values (arithmetic average).

median–the middle value in a series of ordered values.

medical decision level–a concentration of an analyte at which a medical decision is made in the interests of the patient.

mode–the most frequently occurring value in a set of values.

negative predictive value of a test–the likelihood that a patient with a negative test for a disease does not have the disease.

nonparametric statistics–statistics used when the assumption of a Gaussian distribution of the data is not valid.

outlier–a value that is significantly beyond the range of all other values in a set of data; the outlier value is assumed to be from a population other than the one sampled.

parametric statistics–statistics used when the assumption of a Gaussian distribution is valid.

positive predictive value of a test–the likelihood that a patient with a positive test for a disease has the disease.

precision–the random variation (error) in a set of replicate measurements.

proportional systematic error–a systematic error that is proportional to the concentration of the analyte.

quality assurance program (laboratory)–a system of goals, policies, and laboratory activities to monitor the quality of testing processes, identify and correct problems, and ensure accurate and precise test results and competency of laboratory personnel.

random error–error that affects the precision or repeatability of a laboratory procedure. It is the error observed when one property of the same sample is repeatedly measured.

range–the difference between the smallest and the largest of a set of values.

reportable range–the concentration range of a laboratory procedure within which the accuracy and precision are sufficient for medically valid test results.

standard deviation *(sd)*–a measure of variation around the mean in a group of values, calculated as the square root of the variance.

standard error–a measure of the variation in a population, estimated by dividing the standard deviation by the square root of the number of values in the set of data.

systematic error–nonrandom error or bias that affects the accuracy of a laboratory procedure; the difference between the measured amount of an analyte and the true amount.

target mean–the mean value established for each analyte in a control material.

total analytic error–an estimate of the error that could occur with any single measurement on a laboratory procedure; the aggregate of the systematic and random analytic errors of the procedure.

usual standard deviation–an estimate of the precision that a laboratory procedure can achieve; the average of several periodic standard deviation values based on the quality control values in each run of the procedure.

variance–a measure of the distribution of values in a population; the square of the standard deviation.

References

1. US Department of Health and Human Services. Medicare, Medicaid, and CLIA programs: regulations implementing the Clinical Laboratory Improvement Amendments of 1988 (CLIA). Final rule. *Fed Regist* 57: 7003–7288, 1992.

2. International Organization for Standardization. Quality management and quality system elements. Part 2. Guidelines for services. ISO 9004–2: 150, 1991. Geneva.

3. Westgard JO, Carey RN, Wold S. Criteria for judging precision and accuracy in method development and evaluation. *Clin Chem* 20: 825–833, 1974.

4. Tonks D. A study of the accuracy and precision of clinical chemistry determinations in 170 Canadian laboratories. *Clin Chem* 9: 217–233, 1963.

5. Tonks D. A quality control program for quantitative clinical chemistry estimations. *Can J Med Technol* 30: 38–54, 1968.

6. Cotlove E, Harris EK, Williams GZ. Biological and analytical components in long-term studies of serum constituents in normal subjects. III. Physiological and medical implications. *Clin Chem* 16: 1028–1032, 1970.

7. Ehrmeyer SS, et al. 1990 Medicare/CLIA final rules for proficiency testing: minimum intralaboratory performance characteristics (CV and bias) needed to pass. *Clin Chem* 36: 1736–1740, 1990.

8. Westgard JO, Burnett RW. Precision requirements for cost-effective operation of analytical processes. *Clin Chem* 36: 1629–1632, 1990.

9. Westgard JO, Klee GG. Quality management. In *Teitz Textbook of Clinical Chemistry*, ed. CA Burtis, EA Ashwood. WB Saunders, Philadelphia, 1994.

10. Westgard JO, et al. Concepts and practices in the selection and evaluation of methods. *Am J Med Technol* 44, 1978. Part I, Background and approach, 290–300. Part II, Experimental procedures, 420–430. Part III, Statistics, 552-571. Part IV, Decision on acceptability, 727–742. Part V, Applications, 803–813.

11. Cornbleet PJ, Gochman N. Incorrect least-squares regression coefficients in method-comparison analysis. *Clin Chem* 25: 432–438, 1979.

12. American Society for Testing and Materials. ASTM Standard E178-68: standard recommended practice for dealing with outlying observations. Philadelphia, 1968.

13. Boyd JC, Lacher DA. The multivariate reference range: an alternative interpretation of multiple profiles. *Clin Chem* 28: 259–265, 1982.

14. Bellamy JEC. Medical diagnosis, diagnostic spaces, and fuzzy systems. *J Am Vet Med Assoc* 210: 390–396, 1997.

15. Bellamy JEC. Fuzzy systems approach to diagnosis in the post-partum cow. *J Am Vet Med Assoc* 210: 397–401, 1997.

Index

AAVLD (American Association of Veterinary Laboratory Diagnosticians, Inc.), 4, 86
Accuracy, 65
  defined, 23, 63
  diagnostic accuracy (efficiency), 69, 70
  quality goals for, 11–16
  recovery as a measure of, 65
  systemic errors and, 23, 28
Allowable error, 12–13, 23, 62, 67
American Association of Veterinary Laboratory Diagnosticians, Inc. (AAVLD), 4, 86
American Society of Veterinary Clinical Pathologists (ASVCP), 4
American Type Culture Collection (ATCC), 45
Analytic error, 11–12, 23, 62
Analytic sensitivity, 64
Anticoagulants, 47
Archives, 54–55
ASVCP (American Society of Veterinary Clinical Pathologists), 4
Atlantic Veterinary College, 13, 85
Audits, internal, 33, 34–35
Avian leukosis, 86

Bacteriology. See Microbiology
Bayesian logic, 59
Benchmark, 13, 16
Between-day variations, 62
Between-run precision, 66
Between-run variations, 62
Bias, 11, 13, 67
Biological variation, 46
Blood gas analysis, 49
Blood smear evaluation, 35
Bluetongue virus, 86
Bone marrow evaluation, 82
Budget, 40, 43–44

Calibrators, 31
Categorical measurements, 32–33
  controls and inspections, 32
  external monitoring, 33
  internal audit, 33, 34–35
  internal monitoring, 32–35
  nominal scale, 17
  ordinal scale, 17
Centers for Disease Control and Prevention, 32
Central tendency measures, 19
Centrifugation, 49
Chain-of-custody, 49–50
Chemistry tests, 79–80
Clinical Laboratory Improvement Amendments (CLIA) program, 3, 13
Coagulation tests, 82
Coefficient of variation (CV), 13, 19–20
Collection technique, variations from, 46–48
College of American Pathologists (CAP), 3
Comparison-of-methods study, 66–67
Confidence intervals, 20–22
Constant systematic error, 62, 66
Continuing education, 41, 42
Continuous measurements, 25–32
  calibrators and controls, 31
  control limits and target means, 26
  control rules, 26–30
  definitive and reference materials, 31–32
  error corrections, 30–31
  external monitoring, 33
  internal monitoring, 25–32
  interval scale, 17
  Levey-Jennings control charts, 26–28
  ratio scale, 18
  selecting and preparing materials, 25–26
Continuous quality improvement (CQI), 3
Control charts
  Levey-Jenning, 26–28
  Westgard, 29–30
Control limits, 26

Control rules, 26–30
Controls, 31
    corrective action for rejection rules, 30–31
    histopathology, 32
    limits, calculating, 26
    microbiology, 32
    number to run, choosing, 28, 30
    reference materials, 32
    selecting and preparing materials as, 25–26
    stability of, 26
Conversion of conventional and SI units, 89–90
Correlation coefficient *(r)*, 67
Cost accounting methods, 43–44
Cost per test, 44, 61
Cumulative mean target value, 26
Cumulative mean value, 28
Cyclic variations, 46
Cytopathology, 34, 82

Daniels Pharmaceuticals and Diagnostic
    Products Corporation, 87
Data distribution, 20, 21, 22
Day-to-day precision, 66
Decision levels. *See* Medical decision levels
Definitive methods, 31–32
Detection limit, 63, 64
Diagnosis and testing, 68
Diagnostic accuracy (efficiency), 69, 70
Diagnostic Chemicals Limited (DCL), 85
Diagnostic sensitivity, 69, 70
Diagnostic specificity, 69, 70
Diet-induced variation, 46
Director, laboratory, 40, 41
Distribution of data, 20, 21, 22

EDTA (ethylenediaminetetraacetic acid), 47
Electronic quality control, 83
Endocrine Quality Assurance Program
    (EQUAS), 87
Equine infectious anemia (EIA), 86
Equipment. *See also* Instruments
    maintenance, 42–43
    service contracts, 43
    troubleshooting, 43
Error. *See also* Random error; Systematic error
    allowable, 12–13, 23, 62, 67
    analytic, 11–12, 23
    corrections, 30–31
    detection, 8
Evaluating laboratory procedures, 61–77
    analytic characteristics, 68

        accuracy, 65
        comparison-of-methods study, 66–67
        correlation and regression, 67–68
        interference, 65
        linearity, 64
        recovery, 65
        reportable range, 64
        run-to-run precision, 66
        sensitivity, 64
        specificity, 65
        within-run precision, 63–64
    documentation, 77
    medical characteristics
        medical characteristics of a test, 69–74
        medical justification for a test, 68–69
        reference values, 74–76
    practicality and potential value, 61–62
Exercise-induced variation, 46
External monitoring (proficiency testing), 33, 36

False negative rate, 69, 70–73
False positive rate, 69, 70–73
Financial management, 43–44
Food and Drug Administration, US, 3
Frozen control material, 26
Fuzzy logic systems, 76

Gaussian distribution, 20, 21, 22
Good Laboratory Practice (GLP), 3
Government's role in quality assurance, 3–4

Handling of reagents and supplies, 45
Handling specimens, 46–50
    centrifugation, 49
    chain-of-custody, 49–50
    collection technique, 46–48
    hemolysis, 48
    intravenous fluid contamination, 48
    labeling, 48
    records of, 49
    rejection of specimens, 49
    storage, 49
    transportation, 48–49
Hematology
    internal audit form, 35
    practice laboratory, 80–82
Hemolysis, 48, 80, 81
Heparinized samples, 47
Histopathology, 83
    controls and inspections, 32

internal audit form, 34
Human health laboratory quality assurance, 3, 33

Icterus, 80, 81
Identification
    patient, 52
    specimen, 52–53
Instruments
    electronic quality control, 83
    laboratory information system interface with, 53
    worklist, specimen, 53
Interference, 63, 65–66
Interfering substances, 80
Internal audits, 33, 34–35
Internal monitoring, 25–33
    categorical measurements, 32–33
        controls and inspections, 32
        internal audit, 33, 34–35
    continuous measurements, 25–32
        calibrators and controls, 31
        control limits and target means, 26
        control rules, 26–30
        definitive and reference materials, 31–32
        error corrections, 30–31
        Levey-Jennings control charts, 26–28
        selecting and preparing materials, 25–26
International Organization for Standardization (ISO). *See* ISO 9000 standards
Interpercentile interval, 19, 75
Interpretation of laboratory tests, 56–60
Interval scale, 17, 25, 33
Intravenous fluid contamination of blood samples, 48
ISO 9000 standards, 3, 6

Justification for a test, medical, 68–69

Kurtosis, 20, 21

Labeling specimens, 48
Laboratory facility maintenance, 42–43
Laboratory information systems, 50–55
    archives and data retention, 54–55
    computerized *versus* manual, 51
    entering results, 53–54
    interfaces with analytic instruments, 53
    patient identification, 52
    quality assurance and management, 55

reference values and, 76
reporting results, 54
security, 55
specimen identification and tracking, 52–53
test order entry, 52
Laboratory quality assurance program. *See* Quality assurance program
Laboratory quality manual. *See* Manual, laboratory quality
Levey-Jenning control charts, 26–28
Linearity, 64
Lipemia, 80, 81
Lyophilized material, 25–26, 45

Maintenance records, 42–43
Management, laboratory, 40–42
Manager, laboratory, 41–42
Mandate and mission, 39
Manual, laboratory quality
    budget information, 40
    laboratory and equipment, 42
    mandate and mission, 39
    organization structure, laboratory, 40
    quality goals, listing of, 11
    services, listing of, 39
    standard analytic procedures, 55–56, 59
    table of suggested, 7
Mathematical concepts for quality assurance, 17–24
    accuracy, 23
    allowable error, 23
    central tendency measures, 19
    confidence intervals, 20–22
    data distribution, 20
    precision, 23
    scale of measurement, 17–18
    variation, measures of, 19–20
Mean, 19
Median, 19
Medical decision levels, 12–13, 16, 58, 71
Microbiology, 83
    controls and inspections, 32
    standards, 45
    variation from technique of specimen collection, 46
Mode, 19
Monitoring by testing, 68
Monitoring for quality
    external, 33, 36
    internal, 25–33
Multimodal distribution, 20, 21

Nachreiner, Dr. R. F., 87
National Bureau of Standards, 45
National Institute of Standards and Technology, 32
National Reference System for the Clinical Laboratory (NRSCL), 31
National Veterinary Services Laboratory (NVSL), 86
Negative predictive value, 70
Nominal scale measurement, 17, 32
NVSL (National Veterinary Services Laboratory), 86

Ordinal scale measurement, 17
Organizational structure of the laboratory, 40, 41

Parasitology, 82
Patient identification information, 52
Percentile, 19
Personnel
    hiring policies and procedures, 40
    motivation, 42
    performance assessments, 41
    staffing level, 42
    training and education, 41, 42
Point-of-care testing, 83–84
Policies and procedures, 40
Positive predictive value, 70, 71
Practice laboratory
    chemistry, 79–80
    coagulation tests, 82
    cytopathology and parasitology, 82
    equipment, 79
    hematology, 80–82
    point-of-care testing, 83–84
Precision
    day-to-day, 66
    defined, 23, 63
    interpretation of results and, 58–59
    quality goals for, 11–16
    random errors and, 23, 28
    run-to-run, 13, 66
    within-run, 13, 63–64
Predictive value, 70, 71, 74
Preservatives, 47
Prevalence of disease and predictive value, 71, 74
Proficiency testing, 13, 16, 33, 36
Prognosis and testing, 68
Property of an animal, 17–18
Proportionality between methods, 68
Proportional systematic error, 63, 65

Quality assurance program
    American Association of Veterinary Laboratory Diagnosticians, Inc., 4, 86
    components of, 4–5
    costs, 8
    Endocrine Quality Assurance Program (EQUAS), 87
    external, 33, 36, 65
    human health laboratories, 3, 33
    manual, laboratory quality, 4, 6–8
    as measure of accuracy, 65
    National Veterinary Services Laboratory (NVSL), 86
    overview of, 4–6
    proficiency testing, 33, 36
    value of, 8–9
    Veterinary Laboratory Quality Assurance Program (VLAQAP), 36, 85
    voluntary *versus* mandatory, 3–4
Quality control. *See* Internal monitoring
Quality goals, 4, 11–16
    analytic error and allowable error, 12–13
    medical decision levels and, 12–13, 16
    proficiency testing, 13, 16
    selecting, 13–16
Quality management, 3, 6
Quality manual, laboratory. *See* Manual, laboratory quality

Random biological variation, 46
Random error, 11, 23
    causes of, 62
    control rules and, 28, 29–30
    regression statistics and, 68
    source of, 30
Random sampling, 18
Range, 19
Ratio scale, 18, 25
Reagents
    handling of, 45
    interfering substances, 62
    records of handling, 49
    testing, 31
Recovery, 63, 65
Red blood cell counts, 80–82
Reference materials, 32
Reference methods, 32
Reference subpopulation, 74–75
Reference values, 74–76
    considerations in developing, 74–75
    defining, 74
    multidimensional, 76
    subcategorizing, 76

Referral laboratories
    chemistry tests, 80
    cytopathology, 82
    hematology, 81, 82
Regression statistics for method comparisons,
    67–68
Rejection of specimens, 49
Rejection rule, 26, 29, 30
Reportable range, 63, 64
Reported value *versus* true value, 12
Reports
    contents, 54
    form of, 54
    standard screening of, 56
Results
    entering into laboratory information system,
        53–54
    interpretation of, 56–60
    reporting from laboratory information system,
        54
    standard screening of reports, 56
Run-to-run precision, 13, 66

Scale of measurement, 17–18
Screening tests, 68
Security of laboratory information, 55
Sensitivity, 64, 69, 70
Serum separator tubes, 47
Serum *versus* plasma, 47
Service contracts, equipment, 43
Skewed distribution, 20, 21, 22
Specificity, 63, 65, 69, 70
Specimen collection, variations from technique
    of, 46–48
Staff. *See* Personnel
Stains, 32
Standard analytic procedures, 55–56, 59
Standard curve, 64
Standard deviation, 13, 19–22, 26
Standards, 45
Statistical significance, 67
Sterility, checking for, 32
Storage of specimens, 49
Stress-induced variation, 46
Systematic error, 11, 13, 23
    causes of, 62–63
    comparison-of-methods study, 66–67
    constant, 62, 66
    control rules and, 28, 29–30

external monitoring programs, 33
    proportional, 63, 65
    regression statistics and, 68
    source of, 30
Système International (SI) units, 89–90

Therapeutic drug analysis, 83
Total allowable error, 16
Total analytic error, 62
Total quality management (TQM), 3
Tourniquets and sample variations, 48
Tracking of specimens, 52–53
Training programs, 41, 42
Transportation of specimens, 48–49
T-test statistic, 67
Turnaround time goals, 13

Units, conversion of, 89–90
Usual standard deviation, 13, 26, 58

Variable, 18
Variation, measures of, 19–20
Variation, sample
    cyclic, 46
    diet-, stress-, and exercise-induced, 46
    from hemolysis, 48
    from intravenous fluids, 48
    random biological, 46
    from technique of collection,
        46–48
Veterinary Laboratory Quality Assurance
    Program (VLAQAP), 36, 85
Veterinary quality assurance programs. *See*
    Quality assurance program
VLAQAP (Veterinary Laboratory Quality
    Assurance Program), 36, 85
Voluntary *versus* mandatory quality assurance
    procedures, 3–4

Warning rule, 29
Westgard control chart, 28–29
Westgard Multi-Rule Procedure, 28–29
White blood cell counts, 81–82
Within-run precision, 13, 63–64
Within-run variations, 62
Worklist, instrument, 53